The Natural Way to Health and Beauty

(Abridged Version)

By Toni DeMarco

Originally published as *The California Way to Natural Beauty*

HEALTH BOOKS
GROSSET GOOD

PUBLISHERS • GROSSET & DUNLAP • NEW YORK
A FILMWAYS COMPANY

A Note to the Reader:

People react differently to dietary and physical variations from their normal routine. We cannot predict how your body will respond to the diets and exercises recommended in this book and, therefore, you may wish to consult with your physician before undertaking any of the procedures described.

All photographs by CHRIS DEMARCO

CONTENTS

CHAPTER ONE

BEAUTY IS A STATE OF MIND

This book puts within your reach the kind of beauty that only a healthy body and healthy mental attitude can give—a lasting, glowing, and growing beauty that will make you someone special no matter where you live or what your age. A lifetime of research has gone into this that will save you time and energy if you are willing to apply what you learn here.

Perhaps you are tired of trying out all the old cliché beauty hypes. You should be; I certainly am. But I am here to lead you, first to the understanding that you are only as beautiful as you imagine yourself to be and, secondly, to tell you all of the physical tools that will inspire you. Having been a model for many years, I can tell you truthfully that a perfectly ordinary looking girl can be transformed into an exquisite beauty in front of a camera just because for that moment she is made to believe that she really *is* beautiful.

Some people, men and women alike, are born with all the right physical equipment to be "beauty stars" in the eyes of the world. But they lack that one precious little thing that it takes to be a real beauty—the consciousness that they *are* beautiful. Conversely, I'm sure that you have seen, as I have, people with seemingly impossible physical shortcomings who nevertheless hold you spellbound with their magnetic beauty every time you have the pleasure of seeing them. This is what I mean by beauty is a state of mind.

This kind of beauty appeals to me because it goes much deeper than skin level. It is the kind of beauty that comes from being happy to be alive. My mother used to say that beauty is only skin deep, but to me, the skin just reflects what goes on deep inside, beyond the physical workings of the body, all the way into the most remote regions of the subconscious.

Of course you are limited by your genetic heritage somewhat (and I have heard that sometimes even this can change too), but within the bounds of your physical limitations there is a whole range of possibilities of which you may have never dreamed. If you have been conditioned all your early life by your parents to believe either that you are not beautiful or made to feel not beautiful, then you will probably go on the rest of your life feeling this way—unless you learn to recondition yourself. Ask any psychiatrist, he will tell you that you are only as beautiful as you feel.

If you could at this very minute confront yourself in the mirror and say that you now see that you are beautiful and really believe it, you would see a transformation before your very eyes. You would see something happen from inside, from behind your eyes. You would see the muscles of your face begin to relax. You would see an inner glow permeate your whole countenance. You actually would *be* beautiful.

But what if you just couldn't find anywhere in you even the remotest little trace of beauty? I rather doubt this because everyone has *something* about them that is beautiful. But what if you couldn't anyway? What would you do then?

Here is where the physical action comes in. For every mental thought you ever had there is a corresponding physical development which includes, of course, your whole body. Your body actually does grow and conform to the mental commands that you give it and have been giving it all your life, even if on a subconscious level. Even the food you eat and the amount of rest and exercise you get is first determined by your own mental wishes for either the way that you want to look or simply expect to look.

Because the physical is simply an extension of the mental (just as a tool is the extension of your hand and arm), you use the tools of good nutrition to improve yourself physically and at the same time you will begin to effect a change in your mental attitude. As you begin to look and feel healthier and more beautiful your mental conditioning will begin to accept it and after awhile the two will work together.

The idea is to develop a "consciousness of beauty": to be conscious of every time that you feel beautiful. If you have never consciously tried to change something before, the task may seem insurmountable. But when you are experienced at changing or developing consciousness, you know that eventually you will have built what you set out to do if you just keep at it.

Your subconscious doesn't really care if what you program into it is entirely true or not; it has only the emotional impact of what you feed it to register. If you can put real belief into saying "I am beautiful," even if you only believe it for a moment, then your subconscious registers "I am beautiful." That is all that matters. Eventually you will have a whole solid structure built of "I am beautifuls" which will have long since pushed aside all the "I am not beautifuls" that you put there before.

This building process will be easy for you at times and difficult at other times, but the important thing is to stick with it and be patient with yourself. Remember, if you have spent a lifetime developing a negative consciousness about yourself, it may take time to change. Especially if you have one of those days when just everything seems to go wrong. But these are the days when you can really accomplish the most if you are aware that you are actually stopping a pattern by refusing to go "on a bummer." The more you reject the notion that things go wrong, the better.

The best approach is to take something negative and change it into something positive. Even if you can't find anything good in a bad situation at least you can take solace in the fact that every experience contributes to your development: a bad experience can teach you a very important lesson. I always tell myself that everything happens for the best. I don't reinforce negative experiences.

CHAPTER TWO

BEAUTY ONLY THROUGH A CLEAN INNER SYSTEM

The Hunzas are a totally isolated microculture of people living in the Himalayas in the northwest part of India. They aren't vegetarians but they have a primarily vegetable diet and lead very active, simple lives. The Hunzas are a favorite example of perfect health and longevity: they have no crime or disease and usually live longer than a century.

Before I did any research about the Hunzas, I had visualized a primitive race of people with little education about health. To my surprise, I found that they were not always the way they are now. Over the years they developed a method of mind control to relax the nervous system, a diet concept which is so pure that there is no room for unnatural foods, active participation in yoga and other exercise, fasting to keep a pure system, investing in health through organic renewal of their soil, and a philosophy of positive thinking that puts love above all else. I would say that all that is quite sophisticated, wouldn't you?

We Americans who are supposed to be so smart still haven't figured out even half of what the Hunzas take for granted as a way of living. But, perfect as it sounds, I would never exchange my way of life for theirs. It just simply could never work for me because I am so conditioned to the pace and variety of our modern society. True, I could drop out and go live in the Himalayas and adapt their lifestyle, but I know I could never be happy there for any length of time. I have found, though, that you can convert what they have to our way of life and reap the benefits of both.

Some of the best things the Hunzas have going for them are the natural limitations of the surrounding country and climate. Since they are virtually cut off from the rest of the world, the only food they have is that which they grow themselves. They never have to worry about getting chemicals, poisons, or mineral-, vitamin-, and enzyme-depleted foods. If Americans were unable to get refined and preserved foods, we would be a much healthier group of people. The topography of the Hunza region is rocky and mountainous which keeps them very active physically in order to grow and get enough food. This insures plenty of exercise and fresh air and eating frugally in the winter months, which, as we are rapidly discovering, is great for health and the figure. They have excellent water containing an abundance of minerals necessary for the body's chemistry.

I suspected that if they were so together in the diet and exercise areas, they would also be mentally alert and receptive to the universal flow of things. If you really get it together in one area, then one after another, the other aspects of your life will easily fall into place. In the case of the Hunzas, their mental and spiritual development is almost inevitable: having a superbly strong, healthy body provides the nourishment for a mind so it can function at its most relaxed and proficient level. You can't take a human being apart, body from the mind, and expect life to remain. Everything about a human being is totally interrelated and one part cannot function without another. If you feed your body you automatically feed your mind and spirit. The more aware you are of everything that goes into making up your whole being, the faster you will develop as a person and the more perfect you will become.

As we are mainly concerned with the proper digestion, absorption, and elimination of food, I will leave a lot of basics about nutrition for later in the book, but keep in mind that all these things are interrelated and in real life these functions cannot be segregated. In the next chapter I will discuss how to be thin and healthy, but first a thorough knowledge of how to keep a clean inner system is necessary. Once the system gets into the rhythm of having a natural, unobstructed flow, then weight control is no longer a problem: your weight just naturally normalizes at what is right for you.

One of the best lessons for maintaining a clean inner system that can be learned from the Hunzas is to keep relaxed through the proper balance of rest, exercise, and a relaxed mental attitude.

Food will not digest nor assimilate properly if you are uptight. Although to do this subject justice, I would have to write another complete book, there are a few relevant points I want to make here:

● The Hunzas do not fear growing old. This is just a cultural concept. The people look forward to their later years and why not if they continue to be healthy and vital even into their hundreds?

● The Hunzas have conditioned their thinking to only expect good to happen. This gives them a cheerful, friendly, and cooperative attitude.

● "An open mind is the fount of eternal youth."

● Meditation is practiced for understanding, peace of mind, and the realization of how the ability to love sets you free.

● Only when one has learned how to love can one know complete freedom including freedom from worry. Worry makes you "uptight" which in turn makes your body uptight. The result is that your digestive system clamps up and you become constipated.

● The Hunzas believe that thinking makes it so. So don't entertain the aspects of life that you don't want to see materialize.

● Music is an integral part of the Hunzas' life as they believe that it rests the mind.

● Overworking or underworking causes boredom but work combined with recreation gives balance and a fresh approach to life.

● Worry induces heartburn, nausea, loss of appetite, weight loss or gain, diarrhea, pimples, hives, rashes, and nervous breakdown. Extended worry causes high blood pressure; ulcers; and rheumatic, cardiovascular, and renal diseases.

● A bit of yoga wisdom practiced by the Hunzas is "Live in the NOW!"*

Some of the basics of the Hunza philosophy about food which were more or less arrived at naturally, have been proven, to a great extent, by modern scientific methods. Let's take one subject at a time and discuss how each contributes to proper elimination (each of these subjects will be discussed in greater detail in the following chapters):

1. PROTEIN: Digestible protein goes through the system easily. The indigestible kind doesn't. Yogurt, kefir, buttermilk, whey, sour-dough bread, and other culture foods set up friendly bacteria in the intestines, which makes for easy digestion.

2. CARBOHYDRATES: The natural sugars found in unadulterated fruits and vegetables are easily digested but are of just the right concentration so that they do not assault and overstimulate the pancreas. Natural starch, such as the kind found in potatoes and wild rice, is a complex molecule made up of thousands of smaller sugar molecules and requires a complex digestive process. Because it contains so much sugar, natural starch must be consumed carefully and in small quantities. Carbohydrates that have been commercially devitalized, such as white sugar and flour, lack many essential nutrients and therefore can be quite destructive if used exclusively over a long period of time. Refined starches and sugars overload the pancreas by dumping too much sugar into the bloodstream at one time. Honey, on the other hand, contains fructose which digests slowly, giving energy lasting for several hours. Carbohydrates can be well-tolerated in moderate amounts, especially in the form of fruits and vegetables in the right combination with other foods. But carbohydrates with a heavy starch content should be limited to one serving per meal.

3. FATS: Fats are integral components of cell structure and the fundamental to many hormones. Animal fats (hydrogenated) have fatty acids saturated with hydrogen which make them solid. Plant fats (polyunsaturated) have fatty acids less saturated with hydrogen so they exist as liquids. Because animal fats exist in solid form, any excess can be stored along the lining of veins and arteries, producing serious constriction over long periods of time. Plant fats or oils, so named because of their liquid form, are natural body emollients, lubricating agents, etc. and help prevent edema, skin disorders, and atherosclerosis. Lecithin found in natural oils is a good agent.

4. VITAMINS: Vitamins work by "synergistic action." In other words, it takes a combination of vitamins, all working together, for any one vitamin to be of any use in most cases. Without the proper balance of foods, there will not be total absorption of the vitamins consumed. This is an unnecessary nutritional waste.

5. MINERALS: The right balance of minerals is necessary for the proper absorption of vitamins and minerals essential for the body. Without proper absorption of minerals the glandular balance can be thrown off which affects metabolism and therefore absorption, digestion, and elimination. Muscle tone is affected by proper mineral absorption, without which the eliminative system will not work properly and strongly enough.

*From *Hunza Health Secrets for Long Life and Happiness*, by Renee Taylor. Englewood Cliffs, N.J.: Prentice-Hall, 1964.

6. ENZYMES: Enzymes digest and divide into small molecules the food we eat. Digestion would be impossible without them. They can change fats into carbohydrates and carbohydrates into fats. Enzymes are compound molecules composed of a smaller protein and nonprotein or co-enzyme molecule. The co-enzyme part is usually either a vitamin or a mineral while the specific protein is synthesized by the body according to your unique DNA code. Many different enzymes are produced by the specialized organs of the digestive tract. These enzymes act to disassemble the various complex proteins, carbohydrates, and fats we consume as foods. Enzymes within cells can convert fats into carbohydrates and carbohydrates into fats. All cellular processes are under the control of the various enzymes manufactured according to your DNA code. The enzymes you consume in food are, of course, broken down into their component amino acids and vitamins or minerals in the process of digestion. They cannot pass through intestinal villi into the capillaries or lacteals because they are too large. Prior to their digestion, they may be of some assistance to the breakdown of proteins in the stomach. By the way, papaya, which contains the enzyme papain which can disassemble fifty times its own weight in protein, might be a useful addition to your diet.

7. METHOD OF EATING:

A. Eat only when hungry. Food taken on a full stomach is not digested and interferes with the digestion of the food already eaten.

B. Never eat too much at once. This overloads the system and results in indigestion.

C. Chew your food well, making sure that each bite is properly mixed with saliva for digestion.

D. Don't drink anything twenty minutes before a meal and wait at least one hour after the meal to drink. Excess liquids dissolve digestive juices which, of course, is bad for digestion.

E. Fruits should be eaten either separately or thirty minutes before a meal so that their liquids don't dissolve the digestive juices. Eaten separately, fruits act as a good cleanser to the system (not recommended for over-acid systems).

F. Salt is notorious for causing water retention and should be avoided as much as possible.

G. Sufficient roughage is necessary for good elimination. Including a small amount of bran with meals eases elimination.

Aside from discussion of the diet, there are a few other points I want to make which reflect the Hunza way of living:

1. SLEEP: No one knows just how much sleep one needs, but it is safe to say that between six and eight hours, or whatever amount of time leaves you feeling well rested, should be taken to give the body time to completely digest and absorb the food you have eaten. This process includes feeding cells, tissue repair, and cleansing.

2. FRESH AIR: Fresh air is an absolute necessity, especially when sleeping, as oxygen is mixed with digested molecules to complete the chemical process of digestion and absorption.

3. DEEP AND RHYTHMIC BREATHING: Necessary to supply oxygen and for complete relaxation.

4. DAILY WALK AND EXERCISE: Necessary for good muscle tone, circulation, and oxygen—all important for good digestion.

5. HALF-DAY FASTS: Occasional partial fasts, if your doctor agrees you are in good health, rest the digestive system and give the body a chance to eliminate some accumulated toxins.

It would be pointless to try to decide whether or not the Hunzas' extraordinary health is due to their mental philosophy or to their regime of diet and exercise. I think that it is a combination. You can take what you think you can use and apply it to your own lifestyle. If you do this, what you have to gain is what they enjoy year after year: freedom from disease, mental illness, poverty, crime, and police. They are reported to be the happiest people in the world.

It is extremely difficult to measure the time it takes to digest individual foods because mixing foods can speed up or slow down the digestive process. A meal of ordinary mixed solid and liquid food takes about four hours to leave the stomach.

Even in a mixed meal the carbohydrates are digested and pass through the stomach the most rapidly. The protein foods take an intermediate time—meat in large lumps takes about nine hours but ground beef or liver paté leaves quickly. Fats take the longest time of all—from about eighteen to twenty hours. Meals on the fatty side take about six hours to digest.

Liquids bypass solids and are out of the stomach in about ninety minutes. Let me emphasize once again that liquids with meals tend to dilute the digestive juices and wash the water soluble vitamins out through the intestines before they have been absorbed. A moderate amount of liquid is fine but save most of your drinking for between meals when it is really useful to complete the digestive and eliminative processes.

Just as important as the digestion of food is its elimination. I can't emphasize enough the importance of roughage in the diet to keep a clean, flowing system. Too little attention is given to foods once they leave the stomach and are in the eliminative tract. At this point most of the nutritive value has already been absorbed and what is left is just waste. How quickly this waste food matter leaves the intestines is very important to your health. If you are constipated a great deal you already know how uncomfortable slow evacuation feels. A person who eats a high-fiber (especially high vegetable fiber) diet has well-formed, odorless easy evacuations at least every twenty-four hours, but someone who eats highly refined foods and almost no roughage or fiber-containing foods may take as long as three days (and up to two weeks) to rid himself of a meal and experience much pain as a result.

A high-fiber diet is provided naturally by eating unrefined foods with an emphasis on fruits and vegetables in as close to their natural form as possible (including their skins, strings, hulls, etc.). Adding bran to the diet is useful in making the transition from the normal American highly refined, low-fiber diet to a permanently healthy diet or regime for life which contains a high content of fiber. From one teaspoon up to four tablespoons of bran before or at each meal (depending on how much more roughage is needed in your diet) can be taken with water, juice, cereal, or in any other imaginative way you can conjure up. You will find that a high-fiber diet not only will relieve your constipation after only a week, but that if you ever have had a weight problem, this too will disappear. Not only are low-fiber diets conducive to constipation and obesity, but they have been proven to be one of the major factors in causing hemorrhoids, varicose veins, appendicitis, cancer of the colon, and heart attacks.

CHAPTER THREE

WHAT, WHEN, AND HOW MUCH SHOULD YOU EAT?

A lot has already been written about food combinations and when and how much you eat. This is a very important concept in achieving proper digestion, absorption, and assimilation of foods.

What You Should Eat

The following outline should serve as a guide for your new "regime" for life. This is only a general guide for your overall diet. If you find it difficult or impossible to avoid foods that I say should not be eaten, you can appreciate the extent of your addiction. Your body may crave them as stimulants especially if you are a victim of low blood sugar (hypoglycemia). So, just like a junkie trying to break the drug habit, you may have to cut down a little at a time. Don't be too harsh on yourself. Just the awareness of what foods do in your body will gradually make you *want* to eat better. Don't expect to do it all at once but be persistent. Don't punish yourself either. If you need to splurge once in a while it might be good for your head. Just splurge *small* if you feel you must. And SMILE!

A Regime for Life with Special Emphasis on Getting and Staying Slim

Basic Good Foods (Eat exclusively for from one to three months to cleanse or to decrease weight.)

Alkaline-Forming Foods

Leafy, green vegetables such as romaine and red-leaf lettuce, watercress, spinach, beet and mustard greens, kale, and bok choy (raw or steamed)[1]

Other vegetables with low-starch content like tomatoes, cucumber, carrots, long-neck yellow squash, zucchini, string beans, broccoli, asparagus, beets, fresh green peas, okra, eggplant, onions, cabbage, peppers, mushrooms, and artichokes (raw, steamed, or baked)

Fresh fruit, especially papaya, and including peaches, pears, apples, oranges, grapefruit, melon, mango, kiwis, berries, cherries, and pineapple.[2] Bananas only if very hungry as a between-meal snack. (Water-packed or frozen fruit only if fresh not available. Stewed or cooked fruit occasionally)

[1] An exception to the rule, beet greens are acid-forming and onions are neutral.
[2] Cranberries, plums, and prunes are also acid-forming.

Acid-Forming Foods

Milk and buttermilk[3] (raw if available), yogurt, and kefir*

Cheese (raw if available) including Cheddar, Swiss, cottage, goat, ricotta, and fresh Parmesan (easily digested).[4] * No processed cheeses

Eggs, especially yolks*

Pumpkin or squash seeds with any of the following: sunflower seeds, ground sesame seeds, Brazil nuts, pistachio nuts, black walnuts, or cashews (or any nut butters or ground nut blends of the same combinations; all nuts best eaten raw)[5]*

Tofu (soybean curd) plus any of the above nuts or seeds (except pumpkin or squash seeds), dairy products, or wheat germ*

Wheat germ plus any of the above nuts and seeds, vegetables, dairy products, or fish*

Fish, oysters, clams (raw, steamed, baked or boiled)*

Lamb, veal, chicken, organ meats such as liver, sweetbreads and brains (all fat cut off meat and meat eaten raw, steamed, baked, or broiled; moderate amounts)*

Yeast (suspected complete in active state), brewer's yeast with milk, spinach, and many other foods*

Whole-grain toasted wafers (no salt)

Neutral

Vegetable oils and olive oil (untreated by heat), lecithin, avocados, and butter

Honey occasionally (raw if available)

Water, tea (especially rose hips), coffee sparingly (if necessary sweeten with honey or an occasional artificial sweetener)

Foods to Add Gradually as Health Increases (If overweight don't add until weight has decreased and stays where you like it. If underweight, add these foods immediately.)

Alkaline-Forming Foods

Vegetables with a higher starch content like potatoes (skin on), cauliflower, wild rice, squash, corn,[6] parsnips, and sweet potatoes (steamed or baked)

Beans including soybeans, mung beans, and black beans

*All of these foods provide complete protein if eaten in the suggested combinations.

[3] Another exception, milk is neutral.

[4] Cheese should only be eaten occasionally and in small amounts because it is fermented and difficult for most people to digest. It is also highly concentrated protein and very mucus-forming.

[5] These are complete protein combinations and should be treated as the meat part of a meal, not to be snacked on arbitrarily. They should not be eaten with fruits or other liquids unless ground or chewed extremely well. Nuts have more calories than the other protein foods listed but this is because of the high content of polyunsaturated fats which are beneficial for the dieter in moderation. Nuts should be eaten only occasionally and in small amounts as they are hard for most people to digest.

[6] Another exception, corn is acid-forming.

Bananas and grapes

Dried fruits such as figs, dates, and raisins

Neutral

Real cream, and up to 25 percent of the day's fat intake in animal fats including butter (avoid aerosol whipped cream)

Acid-Forming Foods

Wheat germ (a complete protein if complemented by grains, vegetables, nuts and seeds, dairy products, or fish)

Grains including wheat (whole, cooked or whole-wheat cream of wheat), rye, barley, oatmeal, hi-pro granola, millet,[7] brown rice, and whole-grain cereals, and breads made from whole-grain cereals

Cream sauces or gravy made with whole-wheat flour (blended with two tablespoons of soy flour per each cup whole-wheat flour) or other grain flours

Spaghetti or other noodles made with whole-wheat or soy flour

Beef, rare or raw in small amounts

Eat Only Occasionally Once Desired Weight Reached

Neutral

Homemade honey ice cream

Fruit jam made with honey

Hot chocolate

Acid-Forming Foods

Sweets made with honey and/or whole-wheat flour

Pancakes and waffles

Hi-protein drinks

Other nuts such as pine nuts, almonds, English walnuts, macadamia nuts, hazelnuts, filberts, and coconut

Dessert cheeses such as Brie, Camembert, and cream cheese

Never Eat

Neutral

Refined sugar[8] in any form including syrup, yogurt with sweetened fruit, sugar-sweetened juices, sweet mixed drinks, liqueur, soft drinks, candy, and commercial ice cream

Alcohol (except for occasional wine or beer or a rare drink)

---

[7] Another exception, millet is alkaline-forming.

[8] Secondary sugar choices when honey not available: raw sugar, dark brown sugar, maple sugar, and molasses.

Salt in excess (almost any salt is excessive)

Acid-Forming Foods

Refined, bleached and/or enriched white-flour products such as cookies, cake, pastries, noodles, white bread, instant cake and muffin mixes, and unbaked premade rolls and cookies

Pork, ham, sausage, bacon, hot dogs, salami, bologna, Spam, and other fatty meats made from waste products

Fried foods such as popcorn, French fries, potato chips, French toast, fried chicken, etc.

Probably Acid-Forming Foods

Foods prepared with hydrogenated fats such as Crisco, lard, cooked or heat-processed oils, and cooked animal fats

Foods containing fats or oils subject to rancidity such as vending-machine roasted nuts and popcorn, and food on store or home shelves for a long time

Foods containing fats or oils subjected to very high temperatures

Packaged foods containing preservatives

Canned foods (if fresh not available, frozen is next best)

Combinations

If you suffer often from indigestion it will probably be a relief to learn that there very definitely is a sequence to be followed when eating which may prevent it. If you think that you are allergic to some foods such as fruit and nuts, you may have a pleasant surprise in store for you; it may just be that these foods weren't taken in the right order or combination. However, you cannot expect instant miracles. I remember my man Chris and the unpleasant side effects he suffered from a too rapid cleansing of his system after years of toxic build-up. Approach this slowly and carefully. If you have suffered or are suffering from chronic digestive disorders be sure to consult with your doctor before making any radical departures from your usual diet.

Fruit seems to be a food which gives many people trouble. Aside from the fact that it is fairly aggressive as a cleanser and is hard for people with weak systems to take, there is no reason why most people can't grow to like it and include it in their daily diet if they learn the proper way to eat it. If you are one of these people or if you do like fruit or have trouble with digestion and constipation, then learn how to combine fruits and other foods successfully for vastly improved health and more energy.

If fruit is to be part of a meal, it should be eaten first because its grape sugar is fully developed and it digests quickly—about fifteen minutes. It takes vegetables considerably longer to be broken down into fruit sugar so they should be eaten fifteen to thirty minutes after the fruit. Even though the stomach has two compartments and can usually separate foods with opposing digestive requirements, it sometimes cannot separate certain fruit and vegetable mixtures which consequently sour and contaminate the bloodstream. The fruits which *can* be eaten with vegetables are apples, avocados, bananas, citrus fruits, pears, pineapple, melon, berries, and papaya. Even so, I personally find that the juicier fruits are better between meals, because they don't leave me feeling bloated. *All* other fruit should be eaten ahead of the vegetables by at least fifteen minutes, and then only in small proportions.

With reference to digestion, the grape sugar must be extracted from fruits and vegetables during digestion. In ripe fruits the grape sugar is fully developed so digestion takes place in almost no time at all. In fact, because a fully developed sugar is a simple sugar which has not been chemically bonded to others in order to form a more complex carbohydrate, it requires no enzymatic chemical digestion and can act as soon as it has passed through the villi walls. However, unripe fruits are still in a starchy state and take longer to convert. These fruits should therefore be baked. Some vegetables, the root variety in particular, can be more easily digested if the grape sugar is developed by cooking them first. The same is true of grains in their dried state. Although you probably won't come across it too often, grains in their green state can be eaten raw as they start out in a state of full grape sugar development. Corn is one of these grains. Christ and his followers were supposed to have eaten grain in this state. Grain's digestibility can be improved by "dextrinization" or toasting lightly in the oven before cooking.

All fruits (except prunes and cranberries) have an alkaline base. In a meal where fruits and vegetables are combined there should be no beans, mushrooms, or grains. Yeasted bread should be avoided with juicy fruits. Cream should be used instead of milk with fruits. Baked or dried fruits should be taken after the meal. Strawberries should never be eaten with citrus fruits because of their opposing acids. Nuts should not be eaten with juicy fruits unless they are ground or in butter form or unless particular care is taken to chew them very well.

Citrus fruit alone acts as an eliminant. By the way, citrus fruit is alkaline-forming although many people think it is acid. It may have an acid reaction if combined with the wrong foods.

Sweets, especially taken on an empty stomach, create a very acid basis which overloads the system. An occasional sweet properly combined with other foods is good as it forms alcohol sometimes necessary for digestion. Two or more starches in a meal should be avoided.

Starch and beans are a good combination, however. Also exceptions are combining grains and combining different kinds of beans.

Some people avoid nuts because they seem to be indigestible; however, if they are eaten in very small amounts, chewed well, and not eaten with liquids (or fresh fruits) they assimilate very well in a healthy digestive system. Nuts can be finely ground in a blender for use in foods and nut butters and "creams" are another good way around this problem. Nuts should never be subjected to high temperatures as this makes them indigestible, but baking them in a moderate oven is fine. Nuts should not be combined with cheese, eggs, mushrooms, or beans.

All vegetables (except Brussels sprouts, legumes, and rhubarb) are alkaline-producing. Root vegetables are closer to the acid side of an acid/alkaline scale than the leafy green ones. Beans should not be eaten with eggs, fruit, or mushrooms.

Some people find that mushrooms should not be eaten with cucumbers, eggs, eggplant, fruits, okra, beans, spinach, tomatoes, and sprouts but I have never had any problems with these combinations.

Some nutritionists advise against mixing milk and citrus fruits while others suggest that milk is made more digestible by the addition of a bit of lemon juice. The combination of milk and orange juice is even suggested as a tonic. I will leave this one up to experimentation on your part. Another indigestible combination is coffee and milk but cream is okay as it doesn't produce acidity. At any rate, coffee should only be taken black after a meal and only a very small amount if taken within the first hour.

Combining Liquids with Foods

It is generally agreed that drinking a lot of liquid during a meal obstructs digestion, so it is a good idea to wait thirty minutes before and after a meal before drinking. This includes soup . . . better eaten alone. Also it is better to take fruit first in a meal and wait a few minutes for digestion before continuing. If you prefer fruit afterward, wait two hours, so the liquids from the fruit don't dilute the digestive juices. Otherwise, you should drink as much liquid as you want—the more the better for cleansing between meals.

When You Should Eat

Eating should be in tune with your body's cycles: there are times in the day that are natural periods to eat, and there are other times that are natural periods to fast. If you haven't done so already, once you have trained your body to recognize these cycles you no longer have to think about when to eat but do so automatically. And, just as there are daily cycles, there are yearly cycles which require increasing and decreasing food intake according to your body's needs.

If you allow this sensitivity to cycles to extend a bit further, it will also become second nature for you to "feel" which food combinations are right for you, or at least be able to recognize when they are wrong according to how you feel after you have eaten them.

There are nutritionists who advocate the very popular theory of eating "breakfast like a king, lunch like a queen, and dinner like a pauper"* but this is not necessarily a good rule.

But perhaps you have never thought about when you should eat, taking for granted that you eat three meals every day at more or less the same times. What if you're not hungry? Should you eat anyway? Especially at breakfast when you know you *should* eat but just can't seem to make yourself do it. Or what if you are a real trooper and you go ahead and eat breakfast anyway because you think it's good for you?

By now I'm sure you know what I have to say about that: Your own instincts are usually the best. In the whole animal kingdom, there is no animal that will eat when it is not hungry. It is also instinctive for an animal to fast when it is sick until it gets well.

Let me tell you about my daily system of eating: I find that what works best for me is to have yeast broth or a little apple juice or fruit when I awaken or a bit later two poached eggs or a fruit "smoothie" (which includes one or two raw egg yolks, one half cup apple juice, one half cup water, one piece of fresh fruit such as a peach, and one half teaspoon vanilla. The egg has just enough protein to keep me going for a couple of hours. Milk or kefir can be used instead of water). Then when I get hungry two or three hours later I usually have a light meal

*Adelle Davis, who recently died of cancer, was a main proponent of this philosophy. The typical hypoglycemia diet insists on a high-protein breakfast and diet but this can cause other abnormalities.

consisting of a salad, fruit or an open-faced sandwich and make sure to include a small amount of a complete protein like chicken or fish.

Four or five hours after lunch I either have a light snack or dinner, depending on my plans for the evening. If I choose a snack I usually eat dinner two or three hours after that. In between meals if I'm hungry I might have fruit juice diluted with spring water or natural sparkling water or fruit or dried fruit such as a fig or two. Or if I'm just thirsty I have a glass of water or a diet soda (don't overdo these though because of artificial sweeteners).

A smart idea for good health is what I call a half-day fast (unless you are under a doctor's care or taking medication—then you'd better check with him or her first). It is best to start this partial fast in the morning because the body has already had a good six or eight hours start in the process of the elimination of waste. As soon as you start eating, your body must switch from the job of elimination to that of digestion. It is very healthy for the body to be able to cleanse itself of any wastes, acids, toxins, and drugs that have been accumulating for most of a lifetime. When this is accomplished, the body operates much more efficiently and with increased vitality. A partial fast turns back the hands of time as well as beginning a cure for every illness there is. A fast will only be as effective as your diet is when you resume eating again. Just make sure that when you get hungry that something nourishing with a little protein is on hand (a "smoothie" is ideal) for energy that lasts until your first meal.

Longer fasts accomplish the same thing much faster but they can be very dangerous unless conducted by an expert. A fast can only be possible if preceded by a long, cleansing preparation diet.

Everyone in good health can benefit from a partial fast. The best evidence for this argument is to listen to what your body tells you. I am never hungry when I first get up. Not being hungry is normal, but if you have been used to eating a big breakfast every morning this might be a hard fact to believe. Try an experiment tomorrow and see how long you can go without eating before you actually get hungry. Even this may be impossible if you are overly breakfast-conditioned. If you were to lighten your evening meal you would probably find that your breakfast appetite would disappear.

A lemonade "tea" (one half a lemon in a cup of hot water) with or without honey would be a good beginner if you are just a bit hungry or thirsty. Or your favorite breakfast drink like apple juice would be good too. Even some coffee would be all right if you think it would help you to adjust to the idea of no breakfast. Even better than coffee would be yeast broth which is especially good for replacement of the B vitamins. This protein drink is easy to digest and is a smooth way to break your fast. Just add one teaspoon granular active dry yeast to one cup of hot water. But be sure to wait forty-five minutes before eating. If you have eaten anything other than milk beforehand, wait at least two hours before taking yeast broth. When you finally get hungry, a light meal of fruit, a "smoothie," or fruit preceding a vegetable salad, and maybe a cooked vegetable dish plus a protein breaks your fast properly by providing a broom for the elimination of wastes that have been loosened in the system and require being expelled.

A half-day fast is also easy for compulsive eaters who tend to be overweight because it gives them the feeling that they are "being good." A heavy meal at the beginning of the day is depressing to someone who eats too much anyway and is a signal to continue eating for the rest of the day. Breaking a fast with a light meal gives encouragement to the dieter as well as actually being physiologically easier on the system and more conducive to getting the day's work done. A good book you can pick up on fasting is *Rational Fasting* by Arnold Ehret.

Let me emphasize my belief: A half-day fast in conjunction with a healthy diet low in mucus- and acid-forming foods will enable you to cure most chronic illness if continued for long enough. It may take a year to see a major breakthrough in your "condition." The idea is to loosen and remove disease-forming obstructions that have been there for a long time.

If you get to the point in your regime where you feel a half-day fast is no longer necessary, wait until you are hungry and have a "smoothie" or fresh, baked, or dried fruit with something like whole-wheat cream of wheat, or oatmeal and fresh cream, or poached or soft-boiled eggs. One of my favorite breakfasts is papaya, banana, and strawberries topped with yogurt, kefir, and a sprinkling of bran and fresh (frozen) wheat germ. Heavy, starchy, and high-protein breakfasts cause excess stress on the organs and make starting your day difficult.

At this point it might be interesting for you to discover how long it takes the body to digest certain foods. Food, except fruit, generally stays in the stomach three hours, then goes to the duodenum for six or seven hours, and then travels to the large intestine for ten to twenty hours. Forty-eight hours after eating, one eliminates most of the unusable waste. The liver, which manufactures bile to digest food, can be stimulated to increase the production of bile with lemonade tea.

Study the chart below to see how long it takes to digest some sample foods:

Time for Digestion

Rice, boiled	1 hr.
Raw milk	2½ hrs.
Hard-boiled egg	3½ hrs.
Whole-wheat bread	3½ hrs.
Boiled carrots	3¼ hrs.
Boiled beets	3¾ hrs.
Boiled cabbage	4½ hrs.
Meats (in chunks)	9 hrs.
Fats	18–20 hrs.

You should wait between meals to give your system a chance to begin digestion. Fruit takes the least time, usually thirty minutes to one hour. Eating between meals is very harmful because digestion may still be in process or your stomach may be taking a needed rest. If you eat between meals it is going to have to work two or three hours more and maybe contend with undigested food already in the stomach and have to deal with yet another combination requiring different enzymes and digestive juices.

How Much You Should Eat

Knowing how much you need to eat will become second nature to you once your senses are tuned to listening to what your body tells you. In fact, your whole system will benefit immeasurably by an open-minded attitude and positive physical action.

So much of what the average person eats just isn't needed by the body. The body then must work overtime to compensate for the overload. Simply eating less, especially of protein, starchy, and "gooey" foods will greatly alleviate the work that the system has to perform.

The fact that you feel compelled to eat more than you need isn't really all your fault. Americans are consumer oriented: They are besieged day and night on TV and in advertising from all media to buy and eat every conceivable kind of junk that can be attractively packaged and pawned off as "food." People are also continuously reminded that they have a nutritional need for this or that vitamin, "enriched" bread, breakfast food, or high-protein additives while nothing could be further from the truth. As if this wasn't bad enough, they also push drugs on the public as being harmless or a safe means to dispel all the ills that result from being an undernourished but overfed public. Sadly enough, drugs don't really do anything but alleviate the symptoms in one area and add to the poisons that the body is already continuously trying to expel. Drugs should only be used for emergencies.

You will be doing yourself a great service if you will break the consumer habit. Eat only when you are hungry and buy only what you need. If the public stops buying junk and insists on nutritious foods, manufacturers will have to change. It is up to you as an individual to influence the media; not the other way around!

Another factor to consider in trying to decide just how much you should eat is your age. When you are growing up you need the kinds of foods that build your body, but once the body is completely constructed, adding "building" foods is foolish. Once you have attained your full growth as a young adult, your food intake requirements should diminish appreciably as your body need only replace those cells destroyed through natural aging or accident.

The problem of how much and how often to eat must more or less be worked out by you. Only you know how active you are and only you can gauge how much building your body needs. The individual's constitution and glandular type must also be considered when planning what and how much to eat.

Some people are happy eating only two moderate meals each day and according to Dr. Giovanni Boni, teacher, acupuncturist, and practitioner of homeopathic medicine, this is ideal for fitting into the "acupunctural clock" which reveals that one's system is receptive to food for several hours roughly between 10 AM and 2 PM and later from around 6 to 9 PM. Of course the times vary depending on what time you sleep and arise. The periods when you shouldn't eat at all are to give the system a chance to eliminate the food and attend to other important bodily functions. There are time periods in which I instinctively chose for myself to eat even before I came across this scientific Chinese wisdom. I usually have a fruit snack preceding my meals by an hour or sometimes less, and this perfectly corresponds to when I am in the absorption part of my cycle.

It is possible to eat four or five small meals in a day, two in each assimilative cycle eaten at the beginning and end. Eating several meals rather than two or three has been suggested for the overweight because it reduces the temptation for overindulgence due to a ravenous appetite. The rest period from eating should be a complete fast but if you feel hungry, diluted fruit juice or fresh fruit is ideal. Even a banana is better than a binge. The evening meal can be early and light if you plan on a late evening meal or snack.

If you are eating good, nutritious foods, this type of eating should satisfy your appetite. Good foods also seem to fill you up faster and hold you up for longer, particularly if you have included lots of salads and raw, starchless vegetables in your diet for bulk. You shouldn't be worried about eating too much if you have the right balance of foods. Eat until you are satisfied but not stuffed. Eating slowly gives you time to figure out when you are really full.

CHAPTER FOUR

RECIPES FOR SUPERNUTRITION

Cooking, for most of us, is something we *have* to do if we expect to eat well and stay healthy. I don't know anywhere in the world where I can find food as nutritious as what we have at home. I decided a long time ago that if I was going to have to live with cooking, I may as well get behind it and enjoy it. The cook who prepares food with love gives an extra dimension to the nutritional properties of the food. Even the most nutritious, expensive foods seem uninteresting and sometimes unpalatable when the cook doesn't really care or resents having to prepare a meal. On the other hand, if it is lovingly prepared, even a meal using the most modest ingredients looks and tastes delicious.

Don't forget, while in your kitchen it's a good time to use isometrics to change drudgery into an effortless body-toning exercise: stand straight—even use your tiptoes. Bend over, keeping a straight back or bend your knees with a straight back to improve your posture. Make every move one of simplicity and grace. It will show in your cooking.

Fruits

Summer Fruit Salad

I like the fruit chopped into bite-sized pieces considerably smaller than you usually get in a restaurant. Some thin-skinned fruits like peaches taste good with their skins left on. (Preparation time, 30–45 minutes; serves 4)

    2 oranges (I prefer Valencia), peeled and cut into small
        pieces (pour extra juice over the salad)
    1 peach, diced
    ¼ cantaloupe or Crenshaw melon, diced or balled
    ½ honeydew melon, diced or balled
    1 banana, sliced thin
    ½ papaya or mango, diced
    5 or 6 finely chopped "White Smyrna" dried figs
    nuts, honey and juice as described below

Prepare and mix together fruits in bowl. Slowly pour honey to taste over the mixture (I usually omit the honey as the fruit is naturally sweet enough); add a few tablespoons of apple or guava juice and a squeeze or two of lemon if you like it juicier. Then sprinkle on sesame seeds or a blend of very finely chopped nuts—for example, walnuts, pecans, and almonds—almost pulverize them in your blender. If you like, mix this with sesame and chia seeds. You can keep this mixture in an airtight container in the refrigerator for when you need it.

Variations: 1. For the dressing try this mix in the blender; some fruit juices or fruit, honey, a few mint leaves, lemon rind, and nuts. Pour over the fruit. 2. Try thinning out a fruit-honey jam like lingonberry or raspberry with fruit juice for a dressing. Or just juice alone. 3. Instead of juice, use a container of plain yogurt sweetened with honey or kefir, a yogurt-fruit drink the consistency of buttermilk. Use any fruits you like and berries in season. I save apples for a meatier salad like a Waldorf.

Fruit Plate with Steamed Wheat and Avocado Sauce

I find this a very romantic plate for two to share in a shady spot on the lawn on a very warm Sunday afternoon. (Preparation time, 50 minutes; serves 2 or 3)

¾ cup hot steamed whole wheat
1 large round of watermelon, rind cut off, seeded, sliced
      into 3 or 4 long spears
½ cantaloupe, seeded, rind cut off, cut into 4 wedges
½ honeydew melon, seeded, cut into 2 wedges, and rind cut off
1 banana, peeled, split lengthwise
1 apricot, halved
2 or 3 whole plums
1 handful of blueberries
1 handful raw almonds

Arrange the fruit on a large wooden plate around a small dish containing the steamed wheat over which is spooned avocado sauce.

1 ripe avocado, seeded and peeled
⅓ to ½ cup yogurt
pinch celery salt
pinch cayenne pepper
pinch cumin powder
pinch curry powder
pinch onion powder up to ½ tsp.

In a medium-sized bowl mash the avocado with a fork while mixing in the yogurt and seasonings until it makes a smooth, thick sauce. (If you don't have yogurt, try sour cream or cream cheese to blend with.)

I follow the rule for cooking grains to steam the wheat: 2¼ cups water for every cup of grain. Add grain after water boils, bring to second boil, reduce heat to low simmer and cook/steam for 45 minutes or until done to taste.

Baked Bananas

I have had bananas baked plain but for a special taste try these. (Preparation time, 50 minutes; serves 3 or 4)

3 or 4 slightly underripe bananas
¼ cup diced orange
1 Tbs. orange juice
1 Tbs. lemon juice
¼ cup brown sugar or honey
1 pinch cinnamon
1 pinch nutmeg

Preheat oven to 325°. Peel the bananas and arrange in glass baking dish. Combine the remaining ingredients in a small bowl and spoon over bananas. Bake, basting twice with pan juices, for 30 minutes or until golden and tender.

Variations: Plain bananas split lengthwise and baked go well as a side dish when the main course is Chinese food, or Cuban and Mexican food. The recipe above would also make a good dessert with these types of foods.

Vegetables

I haven't boiled a vegetable for years. Boiling takes out most of the vitamins, destroys the taste, and makes the vegetables soggy. I've met lots of people who hate vetetables because their mothers presented them with an overcooked, soggy pile of unappetizing, no-taste, colorless stuff and said, "Eat your vegetables, they're good for you." I've had to work very hard to re-educate my husband, but he now loves vegetables. He had seldom tasted anything that hadn't come from a frozen package or a can.

I almost always steam vegetables; otherwise I bake them. I am fortunate to have a pot with an adjustable steaming rack which I got from my grandmother years ago. I have never seen another one like it so the next best thing I can suggest is to buy the metal kind with collapsible wire sides and short legs, which you use in any pot and which costs only $2 or $3. Revere Ware makes a good pot for steaming, although it is considerably more expensive.

Sometimes to reduce baking time, I steam a vegetable first for 5 or 10 minutes just to soften it a bit. Then I bake it in a glass baking dish with a bit of water in the bottom and a piece of tin foil well secured over the top of the dish.

Oriental cooks have another version of the steaming pot in bamboo with three compartments which can all be used simultaneously.

Although I don't do it much myself, the best way of all to preserve the vitamins and juices of the vegetable is to cook it in "Patapar" paper (or cookery parchment), obtained at your local health food store. It only works well with firm vegetables like broccoli and carrots: Cut the vegetables to size, place on the center of the paper, draw up the sides, twist the paper tightly around the vegetables, tie firmly with a string, and submerge the vegetable portion in boiling water with the top out of the water. You may find it useful to hang the package with a string to keep it from tilting and taking in water. The flavor, color, and texture of vegetables cooked this way are well worth the effort. You will have to experiment with cooking time, just slightly longer than the time required for steaming vegetables.

Here are some samples of the time it takes to steam vegetables, cut into large, bite-sized pieces, in a steamer:

Vegetable	Preparation	Time
broccoli	cut 4 inches from top and split into sections	3 to 5 mins.
asparagus tips	topped at 3 or 4 inches	2 to 3 mins.
eggplant	cut ½-inch sections crosswise	2 to 3 mins.
long-neck yellow squash and zucchini	cut ¼-inch rounds	2 to 3 mins.
spinach, kale, and beet greens	center stem removed from leaves	3 to 5 mins.
potatoes, beets, and carrots	cut ½-inch sections crosswise	10 to 15 mins.

Salads

Here are a few tips to remember when making salads:

1. If the salad you are making is the sort that is tossed or is mostly greens, you might prefer to use much larger sized pieces of greens and whole small leaves if they are under 2 inches for freshness and more individual tastes within the salad.

2. The less wear and tear a salad receives the fresher it looks and tastes. For this reason I usually make a salad in individual bowls or on a plate if I am serving four or less people, and never toss. Instead I use the larger pieces of greens on the bottom and build up to the smaller tidbits on top.

3. With the untossed salad, each person serves his own dressing starting first by lightly pouring on a bit of olive oil, then squeezing on the juice of one-half fresh lemon (which has been deseeded), and then spooning a homemade dressing over the top which contains perhaps a base of yogurt, blue cheese, and herbs.

The Everything Salad

Everything but the kitchen sink! (Preparation time, 30 minutes; serves 2 as main dish, 4 as side dish)

½ cup mung bean sprouts, chopped to ¾-inch lengths

6 large romaine leaves, torn into bite-sized pieces

½ medium-sized head "salad bowl" lettuce, torn into bite-sized pieces

1 cup chopped watercress

¼ cup finely chopped parsley

½ cup finely sliced and chopped red cabbage

1 medium avocado, diced into bite-sized pieces

1 small beet, grated (in medium grater holes)

1 medium carrot, grated (in medium grater holes)

1 tomato, sliced in bite-sized pieces

¼ cup sunflower seeds

¼ cup pine nuts

⅛ cup imitation bacon bits

In a large salad bowl add the ingredients in the order listed, pour on dressing such as your favorite oil-and-lemon-juice dressing and toss carefully until the lettuce is well coated.

Variations: This salad tastes just as delicious without the grated beet and carrot, and/or nuts.

You can add or subtract as you please. Try adding capers or chopped artichoke hearts marinated in oil.

The Nucleus (Bibb Lettuce and Cottage Cheese)

This is the invention of Rudy at the Nucleus Nuance restaurant in Los Angeles, the forerunner to many health food restaurants which inspired me to learn a new kind of cooking. (Preparation time, 30 minutes; serves 4)

1 small head bibb lettuce

1 small bunch watercress

5 or 10 leaves of red-leaf lettuce

1 cup alfalfa sprouts

1 avocado peeled, seeded, and sliced in wedges

1 pint small-curd creamed cottage cheese

¼ cup sunflower seeds

¼ cup pignolias (pine nuts)

On four dinner plates arrange the lettuces, tearing into bite-sized pieces. Then put a large scoop of cottage cheese in the centers, arrange the avocado wedges artfully around the plates, lightly sprinkle on the alfalfa sprouts, followed by the nuts.

Variations: Serve with a combination of blue cheese and herb-tomato dressings (half portions of each) spooned over the salads.

Other types of greens used can be varied (though I prefer the bibb lettuce as a base) such as romaine, escarole, dandelion, etc.

Another variation is to add a few halved cherry tomatoes, sliced mushrooms, and capers.

Mung Bean Salad

What could be simpler than this salad as a late night snack for a lot of hungry people? (Preparation time, 10–15 minutes; serves 4 to 6)

½ lb. mung bean sprouts
2 large tomatoes, diced in bite-sized pieces
1 large onion, diced in long thin pieces
1 lb. fresh cleaned spinach, torn into 2-inch pieces
1 large cucumber, peeled, cut into ⅛-inch rounds, and halved

Variations: Thin-sliced red cabbage or a large fennel root sliced thin make good substitutions or additions.

Make this a chunkier salad by adding cauliflower, scallions, and mushrooms, leaving out the onions, and using smaller portions of the other ingredients.

The Aware Salad

This salad was first found at The Aware Inn and later at The Source, both restaurants started by Jim Baker. The Source is still one of the best in Los Angeles, or the world for that matter, for serving clean, healthy, fresh vegetables, salad, and other good foods. (Preparation time, 30 minutes; serves 2)

10 large leaves romaine lettuce, stiff center portions removed
2 large carrots, coarsely grated
1 large beet, coarsely grated
1 medium Jerusalem artichoke, sliced or cut into chunks
1 large tomato, diced
⅓ cucumber peeled, cut into ⅛-inch rounds and halved
1 avocado peeled, seeded, and cut into wedges
¾ cup alfalfa sprouts
¼ cup sunflower seeds
10 or 12 almonds
¼ cup pignolia nuts

In two large wooden bowls arrange in layers the above ingredients as they are listed. Serve with your favorite dressing.

Variations: Serve with a combination of oil and lemon juice dressing and blue cheese dressing (half and half).

This salad can be made even more high protein by adding hard-boiled egg and a scoop of cottage cheese.

Grated Salad

Once you get the knack of making grated salads you will never want to stop. The variations and combinations are infinite but you will find your own favorites. It is very useful to have a small table-mounted grater with three different blades: large, medium, and small. (Preparation time, 30 minutes; serves 1 or 2)

3 or 4 leaves romaine, stiff center portions cut out
4 or 5 leaves bibb lettuce
a few sprigs watercress
1 large long-neck yellow squash, grated medium
1 zucchini, grated medium
¼ head red cabbage, grated medium
2 carrots, grated fine
alfalfa sprouts
1 large mushroom, sliced thin
3 or 4 cherry tomatoes, halved
1 scoop cottage cheese

Make a base of torn romaine, bibb lettuce, and watercress on a plate or large wooden bowl and neatly arrange the grated vegetables, one at a time, in layers in the center. Sprinkle on some sprouts and arrange mushroom slices and cherry tomatoes around the sides. Top with a scoop of cottage cheese and your choice of dressing.

Variations: Try sprinkling on sunflower seeds and pine nuts or maybe imitation bacon bits. Try using only one vegetable or experiment grating other kinds of vegetables.

Brown Derby "Cobb's Salad"

If you're ready to do a lot of chopping, you can prepare a real treat. (Preparation time, 30–45 minutes; serves 1 or 2)

5 large green romaine leaves
2 chicory leaves
1 medium bunch watercress
1 avocado, peeled, seeded, and diced in ½-inch cubes
1 tomato, peeled, diced in ½-inch cubes
½ cup chicken or turkey breast, diced in ¼-inch cubes
2 hard-cooked eggs (some white removed), diced in ¼-inch cubes
¼ lb. Roquefort cheese crumbled into tiny pieces
1 large stalk celery, diced very fine
⅓ cup commercial bacon chips or ¼ lb. crisp, finely crumbled bacon

With a large razor-sharp knife, finely chop the first three ingredients together. In a large bowl add the chopped lettuce and all the remaining ingredients. Toss with an oil and lemon juice or French dressing.

Variations: Use your own imagination to come up with substitutes you might prefer. Finely chopped capers or Italian peppers in wine vinegar make a snappy addition.

add the bean sprouts, turn off the heat, and gently mix in the sprouts. Put this mixture into individual baking dishes or a 10-inch square glass baking dish, cover the top evenly with the cheese, and bake until the cheese is melted, less than 10 minutes.

Suggestion: Serve with a big spoonful of cottage cheese.

Mother's Eggplant

This is indescribably good if you like lots of garlic. (Preparation time, 45 minutes, serves 2 or 3)

2 large mushrooms cut in long cubes
¼ cup butter or oil
4 oz. can chopped black olives
3 slices eggplant (sliced horizontally, ¾-inch thick)
¼ lb. Cheddar cheese sliced ⅛-inch thick or less
¾ cup pine nuts

Preheat oven to 400°. Lightly sauté the mushrooms in butter until they are limp (add 1 or 2 Tbs. water to keep heat down). Add the olives and set aside. Meanwhile have steamer pot going and steam the eggplant until just barely limp (check after 3 minutes). Fill the bottom of an oiled, glass baking dish with the steamed eggplant, cover each slice with the mushroom mixture, followed by a layer of closely packed pine nuts. Arrange the cheese over the top. Bake for about 5 minutes or until cheese melts well over the top. Serve with a generous portion of hot, garlicky tomato sauce over the whole eggplant.

Fish and Meat Entrées

The fresher the meat and fish you buy, the better. Fish especially is best if you can get it before it has been frozen. The flavor is always much better. Shrimp is all but impossible to get before it has been frozen, but one way to have fresh-tasting shrimp is to buy it from a fish market rather than packaged frozen. When cooking it, drop it in boiling water, turn off the heat and let it sit for three to five minutes or until it turns pink; then cool in cold water, peel and clean it, and then heat it the last minute.

Fish filets, steaks, and whole fish are best baked or broiled at a low, slow heat. Something like filet of sole cooks very quickly, so check it after ten minutes when baking and if it is no longer translucent and gray but white and flakey, then it is done. A thicker steak like salmon or halibut takes about twenty minutes (ten minutes on each side) under a low broiler flame and ten or fifteen minutes longer baked. Be careful not to dry the fish out when cooking. Baste it every five minutes or so to keep the fish moist.

As I avoid cooking dishes with heavy meats, I will cover the preparation of meat in individual recipes.

When cooking fowl I occasionally leave the meat on the bones so that I can get a lot of calcium from chewing the bones. This strengthens the body and helps elimination. I prefer to cook roast chicken and turkey, etc. at a long slow heat. About forty-five minutes per pound at 275° (a seven-pound roasting chicken cooks for five and a half hours or longer if preferred). A roast bird will baste in its own juices if you put the roasting dish inside a large, brown paper shopping bag and staple the end closed while roasting. The bag can be removed for browning the last half hour if necessary.

When the meat is gone use the bones to boil for soup stock, taking care to cover the pot so you don't lose calcium.

Mary Louise's Shrimp-Crab Mousse

This is so good I remember it from when I was twelve. (Preparation time, 1½ hours; serves 4 to 6)

    1 can condensed tomato soup
    3 packages cream cheese (3 oz. each)
    2 Tbs. gelatin
    ½ cup water
    2 cups cooked, cleaned shrimp
    1 cup cooked, cleaned crabmeat
    1 cup mayonnaise
    ½ cup finely chopped celery
    ½ cup finely chopped green pepper
    1 small finely chopped onion
    2 Tbs. lemon juice
    cayenne pepper to taste

In a large saucepan bring the soup to a boil. Meanwhile dissolve the gelatin in the water. Add the cream cheese and stir over medium heat until dissolved; then add gelatin mixture. Cool to room temperature (in freezer if you wish). Shred shrimp by hand and add to soup mixture; then add all the other ingredients. Pour into a mold and refrigerate until firm.

Suggestions: As this is quite rich, I suggest serving this over a thick bed of watercress sprigs and possibly having another choice to serve as a luncheon.

Uvo Cebilia

I had this once in a pizzeria in Milan and had to keep going back for more it was so good. This can be made in a few minutes with ingredients you are likely to have on hand in your kitchen. Thin-sliced ham or bacon bits can be substituted for prosciutto. (Preparation time, 20 minutes; serves 2)

    ¼ lb. prosciutto torn into 2-inch strips
    ¼ lb. mozzarella or longhorn cheese, coarsely grated
    4 to 6 eggs (I use 4 whole eggs plus 2 egg yolks)

Prepare the ham and cheese in a bowl, break eggs over top, and stir with fork until barely mixed, breaking yolks.

Tomato Sauce
cayenne pepper
one 15 oz. can tomato herb sauce
⅛ tsp. ground oregano
⅛ tsp. basil
⅛ tsp. thyme
⅛ tsp. fine herbs
⅛ tsp. garlic powder or more to taste

Simmer sauce, while adding herbs, until hot. Pour the egg mixture into greased, individual baking dishes (or one large one), spoon the tomato sauce over the top, and sprinkle with 3 tablespoons freshly grated Parmesan cheese. Bake in a preheated oven at 400° for about 7 minutes or until the eggs are fairly firm when center is checked with a fork.

Shrimp-Bean Sprout Chop Suey

I love this kind of food so much I could eat it every night by just switching around the vegetables and protein choices. (Preparation time, 1 hour; serves 2 or 3)

one 4 oz. can sliced water chestnuts
⅓ cup Shiitake mushrooms, soaked, squeezed, and sliced fine lengthwise
¾ cup Chinese pea pods, ends popped off, strings removed, and
    cut in half diagonally if very large
½ to 1 tsp. very finely grated fresh ginger or more to taste
10 large shrimp cooked, peeled, and cleaned
½ cup slivered almonds

Slice and prepare the above vegetables, nuts, and shrimp before starting the sauce.

2 Tbs. cornstarch
¼ cup water
2 Tbs. Shoyu soy sauce or Tamari

Combine in a small bowl and set aside.

2 Tbs. oil (try part sesame oil)
½ cup thinly sliced leeks, or scallions with tops
1 cup celery cut in long slivers lengthwise and then cut in 1-inch pieces.
    Add some chopped leaves for extra flavor.
1 lb. (or less if desired) mung bean sprouts
½ cup fish, chicken, or vegetable stock

Sauté leeks and celery in large heavy saucepan. When the onions and celery are limp and bubbly add the vegetables and simmer for 1 minute with ½ cup of stock. Add shrimp, nuts, and cornstarch mixture and simmer and stir for 1 minute or until sauce thickens and then spread mung bean sprouts over the top. Cover, turn off heat, and serve after sitting for 2 minutes. Serve the whole pot on the table, each person helping himself to as much as he likes. Serve with a separate bowl of brown rice or steamed whole or cracked wheat.

Variations: This dish has many varieties, depending on what you have in your refrigerator. It can be made with or without shrimp or with crab, other fish, tofu, or shredded chicken if that is your preference. There is a wide range of vegetables which can be substituted like steamed broccoli or greens. If you choose a hard vegetable, presteam it.

Other suggestions for variation: any, all, or some of these can be added.

2 thick branches broccoli slivered into clumps that will steam easily
¼ head cauliflower slivered into clumps that will steam easily
2 cups Chinese cabbage cut in 2-inch strips or sliced Brussels sprouts
3 large sliced mushrooms
5 large leaves of fresh spinach cut in 2-inch strips
2 sprigs mint leaves cut fine
1 small bunch of celery root leaves chopped in ½-inch pieces
one 4 oz. can sliced bamboo shoots
1 medium daikon grated fine and served over the top, or grated radish
   or horseradish if no daikon is available

Chicken

The best way to cook chicken, if you have the time to prepare it in advance, is to bake it for a long time at the lowest temperature possible. Preheat oven to 300°, place the chicken in a glass baking dish with the juice of two or three lemons (and their skins too for a real lemony flavor); add cayenne pepper, thyme, and tarragon; a few chopped garlic cloves; vegetable broth and white wine, sherry, or water to cover bottom half inch or so. Cover with a regular brown shopping bag, staple closed. Cook for one hour at 300°; reduce heat to 165° (or as low as possible) and cook for several hours more according to the following formula:

1. Find cooking time required at 350°: for example, 5-lb.* bird at ½ hr. per lb. = 2½ hrs.
2. Multiply this time by 3: 2½ hrs. × 3 = 7½ hrs.
3. Add 1 hour for precooking: 7½ + 1 = 8½ hrs. total

This method is also perfect for turkey without the lemon.

Otherwise, bake at 300° for 30 to 40 minutes per pound.

If you want to add chicken to another dish, it can be cooked quickly by steaming a cut-up chicken for about 20 minutes. Use very little water so that the resulting broth is concentrated and can be used as is or as a base for gravy.

By the way, I never throw anything out, including the bones and scraps from a chicken. They can be put in boiling water alone or with carrot tops, radish tops, celery, pea pods, or other pieces of vegetables you might otherwise throw out, simmered for 30 minutes, and the resulting broth used as a soup stock or for sauces or gravies.

*Anything smaller than 5 lbs. should be cooked one hour less per pound than the total time for a 5-lb. bird according to this formula. The best way to get it perfect is to experiment on your own and check occasionally to see if tender. Even a 5-lb. bird could get too dry if your oven temperature varies from mine so check an hour or two ahead of time.

Quick Baked Chicken

This is unbelievably simple but I've done it so many times that now I believe it. All you need is a couple of hours while it bakes. This recipe can be used for cooking a turkey too. (Preparation time, 2 hours plus; serves 2 or 3)

3-lb. whole chicken ready for frying or baking
3 Tbs. crushed rosemary and tarragon or your choice of spices
a few shakes of cayenne pepper
1 Tbs. garlic powder

Preheat oven to 300°. Remove the package of innards. Place the bird in a glass baking dish and sprinkle it well with the seasoning. Place in a large brown paper sack, staple the end closed after folding it once, and bake for 2 hours. It should come out juicy, succulent, and almost falling off the bones.

If you have longer to cook the chicken, it is even better. The heat should be reduced accordingly. A general rule is to cook 30 minutes per pound at 350°, but for poultry I like to add 15 minutes for every hour and reduce the heat to 300°. If there is time, use the slow-low flame method described previously.

Suggestions: This is great in the summer, especially with whole wheat and soy spaghetti with olive oil and garlic, and mixed-green salad with dandelion. You don't have to spend hours slaving away in the kitchen. If you are watching your weight leave out the spaghetti and have steamed vegetables instead. Every bit as good!

If you use a larger chicken and have leftovers, try making Chicken à la king or Chicken Curry. Use the bones and all the leftover parts to boil for soup stock. Strain and refrigerate the stock and before making soup remove the crust of fat. Freeze the stock you can't use immediately.

Chicken Tandoori (or Red Chicken), New Delhi Style

Don't be scared away by the spices in this marinade because in the end all you have is tender, crispy chicken with a delicate flavor. Double this recipe for a real feast. (Preparation time, 3 hours, plus marinating time; serves 4)

1 tender, medium chicken
3 Tbs. olive oil
Marinade
4 oz. yogurt, whipped with a wisk
¼ cup olive oil
¼ cup freshly grated ginger
2 Tbs. minced garlic
juice of 1 lemon (4 Tbs.)
1 Tbs. chopped tarragon
1 Tbs. chopped chives
1 Tbs. chopped thyme
2 Tbs. cayenne pepper

1 Tbs. ground cardamon
1 Tbs. cinnamon powder
1 Tbs. saffron
1 Tbs. ground hazelnuts
5 bay leaves crumbled
2 Tbs. beet juice (steam 1 medium-sized beet, cubed, in ½ cup water till
    liquid is reduced to 2 Tbs.—about 10 minutes)

Coat the chicken thoroughly with the marinade and place in glass baking dish. (You can cut preparation time in half by using dried packaged or bottled spices.) Cover and leave at room temperature for at least 2 hours and preferably overnight.

Preheat oven to 400°. Remove most of the marinade with a plastic spatula. Mix any liquid that has accumulated in the dish with the olive oil and pour it over the chicken. Roast for 15 minutes at 400° and then reduce heat to 250° and cook for 1½ hours to 2 hours more until done. Test the thick part of the leg with a knife: if the meat is tender all the way to the bone, then it is ready.

Suggestions: When you double the recipe it is better to use two medium-sized chickens. This chicken is good cooked in a paper bag for added tenderness. The chicken bastes itself with its own steam and the paper sack "breathes" to allow oxygen in. Foil or a cover of metal tends to make the chicken tough. Just slip the chicken in the glass dish into a regular brown paper sack, staple the end closed, and leave it until done. Some people prefer to remove the bag a half-hour before the chicken is done to brown to a nicer color but I like it both ways.

Mizutaki

I think of this as a very festive dish, one of my favorite Japanese recipes. It is very much like Sukiyaki with the addition of a rich, creamy sauce with a homemade mayonnaise base. It is also one of the few recipes I have using red meat. Prepared with excellent beef and sliced paper thin, the meat adds a good, light protein balance to the vegetables which are the main part of this meal.

The idea is to cook the meat and vegetables in a liquid over charcoals in a wok right on the table and let the guests serve themselves. They add and cook more of what they like as the meal progresses. Fingers and chopsticks are a definite advantage. When the vegetables and meat are cooked each guest puts them in his bowl with the sauce and adds more as he goes along. If no transparent noodles are used, have a small bowl of rice on the side to mix with. The liquid left in the bowl after everything is eaten makes a great soup finale when a little broth is added from the wok. (Preparation time, 1½ hours; serves 4 to 6)

Sauce
1 egg
2 Tbs. fresh lemon juice
¼ tsp. dry mustard (optional)
1 cup salad oil

Combine all except ¾ cup oil in blender. With blender on high, gradually add remaining oil in a steady stream.

Stir in the following ingredients and set the sauce aside until just before serving, at which time the sauce should be heated on low (don't boil) and served into large prewarmed rice bowls. (Refrigerate if prepared beforehand):

⅓ cup sour cream
2 Tbs. Shoyu soy sauce or Tamari
2 Tbs. sherry, saki, or wine
⅓ cup broth

Cooking liquid

Preheat 2 quarts of chicken or beef broth (or four 14 oz. cans commercial broth) in a large pot. Pour into a wok when it is not quite boiling and just before you are ready to serve the vegetables. Charcoal briquettes can be heated to red hot under your broiler and placed in the wok just before adding the cooking liquid. If you don't have a wok, bring the liquid to a low boil in a large saucepan on the stove before adding the vegetables. Cook from 4 to 7 minutes; serve immediately.

Vegetables

1 bunch green onions cut in 2-inch pieces
½ lb. fresh mushrooms sliced thin (or substitute a few dried mushrooms called "Shiitake" soaked, squeezed of liquid, and sliced in long strips after cutting off the stem)
2 bunches fresh spinach torn in about 2-inch squares
½ lb. fresh tofu in ½-inch cubes (tofu is soy bean curd, available in cans)
1 cup Chinese pea pods
2 cups Chinese cabbage cut in 2-inch strips
one 4 oz. can bamboo shoots, sliced
one 4 oz. can water chestnuts, sliced

Shirataki

Shirataki noodles are translucent threads of gelatinous starch extracted from a root plant. It is dry when you buy it and should be soaked in lukewarm water for 30 minutes or less before using.

Meat

Use 1½ lbs. boneless beef sirloin or filet mignon sliced paper thin. If you don't have your own meat-slicer it is best to chill the meat until it is almost frozen, and then with a very sharp knife cut into slices no more than ⅛-inch wide.

Add the vegetables, Shirataki, and meat, a little at a time, to the broth, and remove with chopsticks or tongs as each ingredient is cooked. The green onions take the longest, about 5 minutes. The meat only takes a few seconds.

Suggestions: Prepare the meat ahead of time and refrigerate. Prepare the sauce ahead of time and refrigerate. Prepare the vegetables but don't cut until 45 minutes before serving.

Quick Shrimp Gumbo

This is made from ingredients you may readily have on hand. It is a meal in itself, quick to make, and very healthy: a lot of vitamins A and C in the vegetables, and shrimp, of course, is a complete protein with B vitamins. The secret of this is to make it as fast as possible to make best use of the vitamins. (Preparation time, 30–45 minutes; serves 4)

1 large minced onion
2½ Tbs. olive oil
3½ tsp. dried, minced garlic, softened in 2 Tbs. water
1 minced red or green bell pepper (double vitamins for the red)
1½ cups chicken stock (can be added frozen)
one 28 oz. can tomatoes, shredded into bite-sized pieces
one 6½ oz. can minced clams and juice
one 6 oz. can tomato paste
2 bay leaves (whole)
one 10 oz. package frozen cut okra (if fresh steamed okra is used add 10 minutes and lots of vitamins)
1 Tbs. cornstarch
1 Tbs. Bako Yeast (optional)
1 Tbs. Tamari
2 Tbs. or enough water to make a thin paste
2 Tbs. cream sherry
2 Tbs. lemon juice
1 Tbs. thyme
1 Tbs. filé (finely ground sassafras leaves)
1 Tbs. Mexican hot sauce (or cayenne pepper to taste, about ⅛ tsp.)
¾ cup chopped parsley
1 lb. or 16 large, cooked, shelled, and cleaned shrimp

In a large, heavy saucepan sauté the onion, garlic, and bell pepper at medium heat. Add all other ingredients up to and including okra (when sauce gets very hot, 6 to 10 minutes, reduce heat to simmer). Make a thin paste of next four ingredients and add to sauce. Add next ingredients as listed, simmer, and serve in warm bowls as soon as the sauce thickens slightly and the shrimp is heated.

Suggestions: Although I prefer to skip the calories, you might serve your guests brown rice on the side. Start cooking the rice first so it will be finished at the same time.

CHAPTER FIVE

EXERCISE, BREATHING, AND BATHING

One of the most important aspects of health, longevity, and beauty is keeping your body active and in tone by exercise. This word, like "diet," is dangerous to use around someone who has systematically avoided having to do exercises for the better part of a lifetime. If you are at all like me, you hate to do anything that is repetitious, but from time to time you may start a new exercise program because you think that it is something you really need. But just as when you're on a diet, the limitations and repetition become excruciatingly boring and eventually you stop and settle back into your workday routine which probably doesn't involve enough activity to keep your cheeks pink. In a way you were right. There is nothing more destructive for the human spirit than continuous repetition.

But there is a way to solve this problem, and all it really takes is a little imagination and a big desire to keep your body in shape, no matter how thin you are. The best way to start exercising is by doing a little bit at a time and be sure to vary your choices.

Exercise is really essential to stimulate circulation in order to keep a proper glandular balance. When the endocrine glands are functioning properly both the mind and body benefit through clear thinking, calmness in situations of stress, and overall smoothly unified functioning of the body.

Exercise stimulates deep breathing which purifies the blood of carbon dioxide. In case you can't relate to why you need pure blood, it might set you on your toes to realize that the major cause of wrinkles and bad complexion is poor circulation which leaves behind toxins and waste matter in various parts of the body.

Smoking, I need hardly mention, does not do anything positive for your body. If you smoke, I am sure you are aware of shortness of breath, coughing, and other unpleasant side effects. I was a heavy smoker for many years. I smoked because I loved to but I hated myself for doing it at the same time. After a long struggle I kicked it and I'm really happy now that I did. I woke up one Easter Sunday on vacation in Rome feeling sick and disgusted with myself for having gone through about three packs of cigarettes the day before. I had been wanting to quit for a long time and this seemed like the perfect moment. I silently swore to myself that I would *never* touch another cigarette. My man, Chris, had privately made an *identical* decision that same morning and we were each surprised to find that the other was not smoking. Although this made it easier for me to quit, I would have done it by myself anyway. The joy of being free from all that smoke and paraphernalia made it worth sticking to my decision. The first three days were the hardest, but after a week I had almost forgotten I had ever been a smoker, and now, several years later, I never even get the urge. I know that I never did need cigarettes and could have stopped smoking years before if only I had known how easy it would be.

There are some days when I am very busy with work that involves running around from place to place. I know that on these days my circulation is getting plenty of stimulation. Maybe too much in fact. On those days I can't wait to get home and take a nice, long, hot, soothing bath. But after my body has cooled down and relaxed, I like to take a few minutes to do some yoga postures to limber up and straighten out the kinks. This is an absolute necessity after a long photo session where I have been sitting in one pose for hours and hours (it seems) with my body twisted out of shape. A few minutes of yoga does wonders to take away all the aches and pains by loosening stiff muscles and getting bones and the spinal column back in place.

Then there are other days when there is either nothing happening or when I spend hours at my desk writing without moving. If I anticipate that this might happen I like to spend from fifteen minutes to half an hour doing yoga when I first get up. Then later in the day I try to find an hour to take a long walk in the hills. Even if I don't find the hour to walk I like to finish the day getting straightened out again with a few peaceful minutes of yoga.

I love dancing, swimming, running, and tennis and do them whenever I get the opportunity, but my lifestyle right now just doesn't allow the time to do them regularly. There is the latent tendency in me to do nothing at all when I'm engrossed with my work, and that is probably just what I'd end up doing, without the flexibility and stimulation that yoga gives me.

I approach yoga, or any exercise for that matter, just like a little kid. If it isn't fun, I won't do it. I like to turn it into play or a dance, letting one motion flow into the next. I have absolutely no set routine or order although there are things I especially like to do so I do them almost every time. I have a book illustrated with photographs of yoga postures that I refer to occasionally to learn new poses or to remember the ones I've forgotten. If something is too difficult for me to do at first, I keep working on it, from time to time, until I can do it without any strain. One of the requirements of yoga is that you never force your body into any posture but let it come to you naturally.

If you have never studied yoga there are books with simple poses that you can buy to get you started.* Yoga that involves only the execution of physical poses and breath control is called *Hatha yoga.* There are several other types of yoga having nothing to do with exercise, one of which is *Karma yoga,* the use of positive action for the good of others. *Bhakti yoga* is similar in that one devotes one's life to a spiritual path. *Raja* and *Japa yoga* go one step further in using mind control and meditation with a *mantra* (a repeated sound) to achieve a state of bliss. The practitioner of *Jnana yoga* seeks loss of the ego in order to gain wisdom. Swami Satchidananda puts all the different types of yoga together in one and calls it *Integral yoga.* You can read more about it and learn the different physical poses (*āsanas*) from the photographs which illustrate his book (the one I use), *Integral Yoga Hatha.*** You may want to take lessons if they are available where you live. But let me emphasize that it is not necessary to take classes to learn yoga; you can get the basics from a good book or two.

*Introduction to Yoga, by Richard Hittleman (Illustrated with photographs). New York: Bantam Books, 1969.
Yoga for Americans, by Indra Devi (illustrated with photographs). New York: The New American Library, 1959.
**Integral Yoga Hatha, by Swami Satchidananda. New York: Holt, Rinehart and Winston, 1970.

Yoga

In addition to yoga I have included a couple of dance exercises in this section, as there are many similarities of movement and position between the two. I have given my own names to some of these poses or exercises and if they are classic yoga I also give their traditional name.

Unless specifically stated, most yoga poses should be held for as long as comfortably possible. Some are repeated several times with pauses for resting. The most important thing to remember is not to push yourself too hard and to proceed at your own pace, gradually building up strength and the amount of time you can hold the poses. I like to move within a pose—swaying, stretching and flexing, and bending the head and extending the tongue when appropriate for subtle exercise of different muscles. Poses should *always* be done on a carpeted floor or a foam rubber exercise mat for greater comfort and safety. Varying the poses you do daily and switching the order eliminates the chance of boredom. Finally, unless otherwise instructed, you should breathe normally—that is with mouth closed, drawing air in and out through the nose.

I have included these nineteen poses because I think they are the best ones for toning as much of the body as possible in the shortest amount of time. There are many other simpler poses which don't require as much concentration and energy but are equally good for specific areas of the body. It would be to your benefit and enjoyment to buy a book of yoga poses and learn them as well as some of the more advanced ones which I have not included here.

I like to warm up first by doing an exercise I learned in ballet class many years ago which I call the Twist. You stand with your feet firmly planted on the floor about two feet apart (or whatever is comfortable for you). Holding the lower half of your body rigid, keep your arms stretched out, palms down parallel to the ground and swing them from one side of your body to the other, allowing your torso to twist as far as possible to the left and to the right. (*See illustrations 1 and 2.*) Once you have gained some momentum, you can hear parts of your spinal vertebrae pop into place if you are doing this properly. This is a good exercise for toning up the muscles in your waist.

ILLUSTRATION 1.

ILLUSTRATION 2.

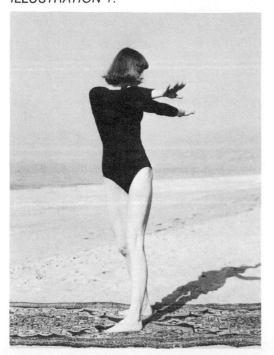

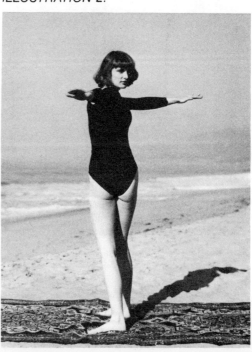

Next you could go into a Back Bend which stretches your body in the convex direction. If you can't get into the bend from a standing position build up to it by lying on your back and pushing yourself up from the floor. But first try doing it standing (feet in same position as for the Twist) by going back as far as you can (arms leading and stretching back) without losing your balance until your hands, palms down, are resting on the ground. While in this position stretch and flex in every direction possible, rock back and forth turning your head as far as you can. (*See illustrations 3 and 4.*) Don't worry if you can't do a full Back Bend because just

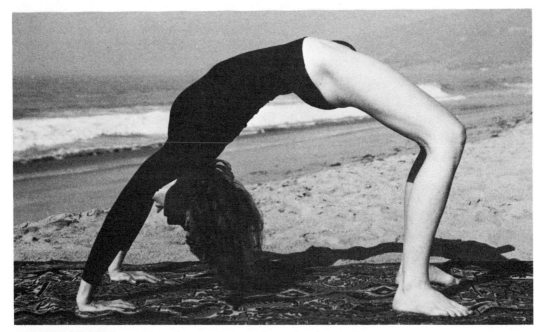

ILLUSTRATION 3.

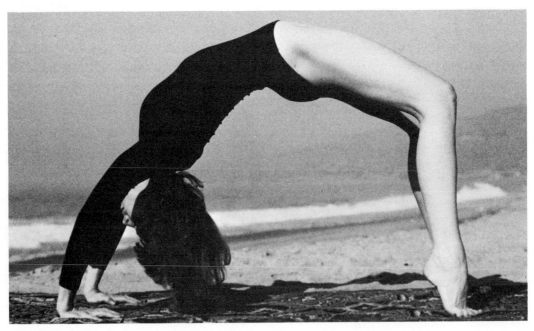

ILLUSTRATION 4.

stretching is an excellent exercise in itself. This exercise is great for the whole body—from head to toe! While still learning the Back Bend you might want to get someone to give you balance and confidence by lightly supporting your back as you bend.

An acrobat could flip over into a concave U from the Back Bend but if you (like me) are not this adept, let yourself down slowly until you are lying on your back with your arms at your sides, legs together flat on the ground in front of you. Then slowly and evenly lift your legs, toes pointed, through to a straight up Shoulder Stand (*Sarvangasana*). You can use your arms, with elbows on the ground, to support you. (*See illustrations 5 and 6.*) This position stimulates the circulatory system. At this point you may want to go into an Upside-down Lotus

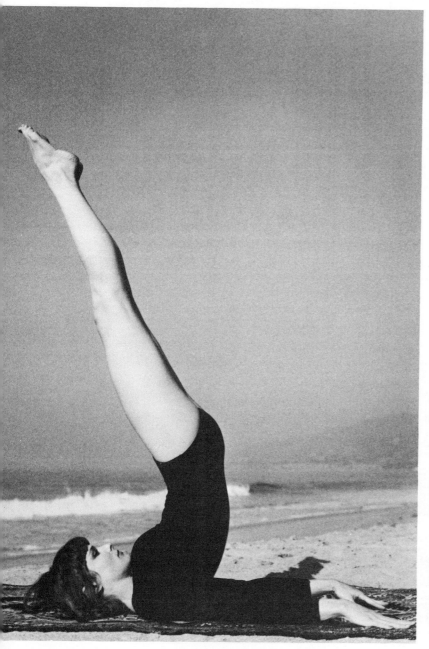

ILLUSTRATION 5.

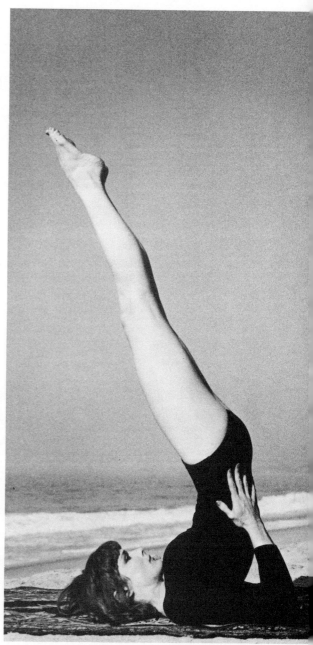

ILLUSTRATION 6.

if you can already do a normal Lotus. (*See illustrations 7 and 8.*) A Lotus (*Padmasana*) consists of sitting with legs crossed and resting each foot on top of the opposite thigh close to the body and resting the hands on knees. For an Upside-down Lotus, cross and hold the legs as in a Lotus while in a Shoulder Stand. Beside being good for circulation, the Upside-down Lotus is an excellent exercise for leg muscles, particularly the inner thighs. Both this and the regular Lotus are recommended as poses for meditation.

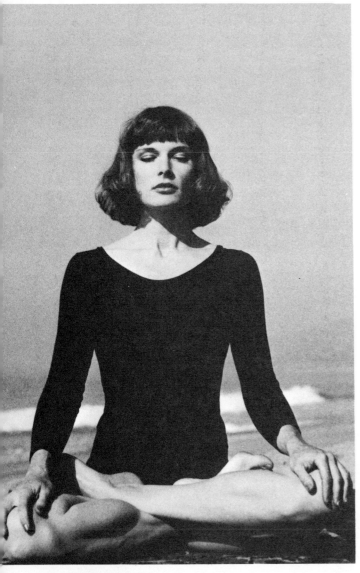

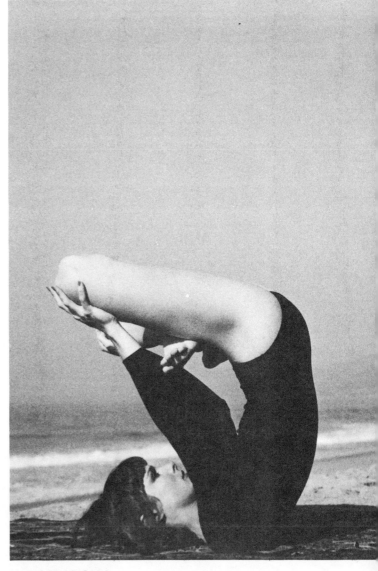

ILLUSTRATION 7.   ILLUSTRATION 8.

If you are a beginner and cannot do an Upside-down Lotus, continue from the Shoulder Stand, lowering your legs all the way back over your head until your toes touch the floor. Then reach back with your arms and grab your toes and stretch and flex as much as you can in the position that I call the Sandwich, first with your feet at right angles to your legs and then with your toes pointed. (*See illustrations 9 and 10.*) Do this for as long as you can stand it. This

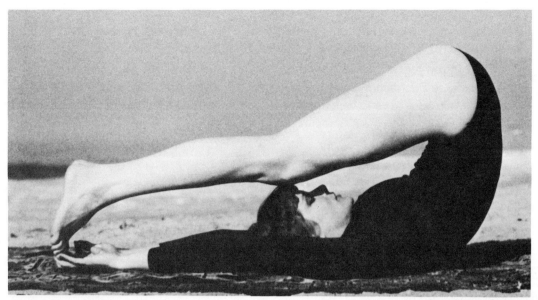

ILLUSTRATION 9.

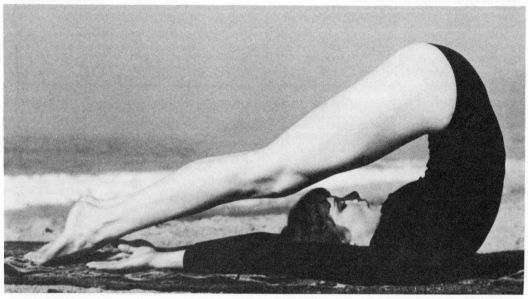

ILLUSTRATION 10.

exercise is great for toning the back of the legs and the thighs. If you find that you're having difficulty, try doing it at the end of the day when you are more limber. As a matter of fact, you will find that all of these poses are easier at night. I suggest taking 10 or 15 minutes in the morning to do some exercises and either repeat or continue others for another 10 or 15 minutes in the evening. If you miss a day or two or only get in 5 minutes don't feel bad because this happens to everyone and it is still infinitely better than no exercise at all.

If you do your exercises in the morning, do them before eating breakfast—that way you won't interfere with the digestive process. Day or night, give your stomach a couple of hours to get the major part of your meals digested so that you will feel comfortable in your yoga poses.

From the Sandwich, if you are limber enough, you can go into the Suspension Bridge (*Bhujangasana*). Leave your feet where they are and bring your arms to your sides flat on the ground, palms down, and slowly push your body backward and roll your head forward. You will end up lying on your stomach with your feet still not having moved, your arms having done all the work. (*See illustration 11.*) If you're not yet this agile, simply let your legs down (as slowly as possible for extra exercise) and roll over. From here lift yourself up by making a

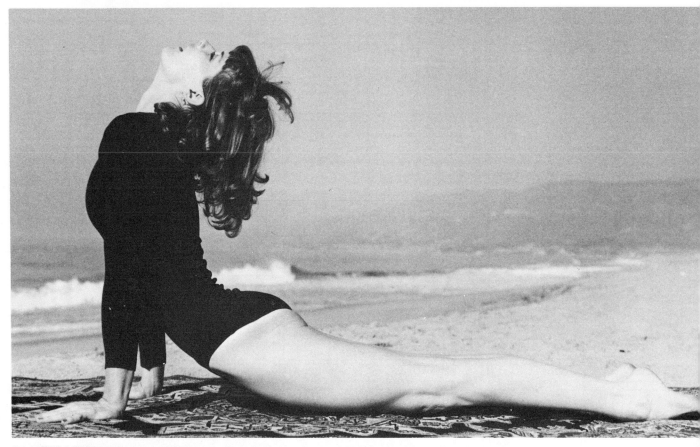

ILLUSTRATION 11.

Suspension Bridge of your arms and leaning forward lift your torso off the ground, using your arms and toes to bring you up. (*See illustrations 12 and 13.*) Now lift your back up in an arch and use your arms to "walk" backward (*see illustration 14*) until your legs are in a standing position and you are touching your toes in a Stand Up Sandwich. Hold this as long as possible, using your arms to bring your head as close to touching your knees as possible. (*see illustration 15*) and then slowly "walk" on your hands back to the Suspension Bridge. Let your back "hang" down as much as possible—you will feel spinal vertebrae slipping into place when you gently jiggle your body in this position. Keep the heels of your feet on the ground and bend your head back as far as possible then stand on your toes, your feet now making a right angle with your legs, and arch your back again. Repeat these convex to concave positions several times. This is a good exercise to relieve back pains and strengthen stomach and leg muscles.

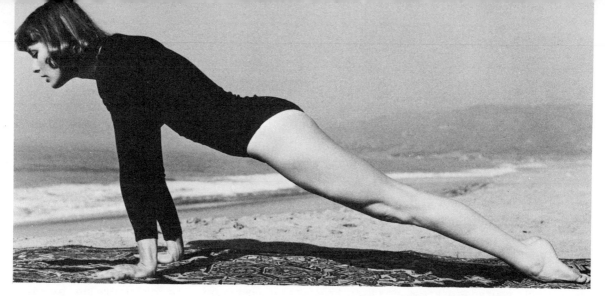

ILLUSTRATION 12.

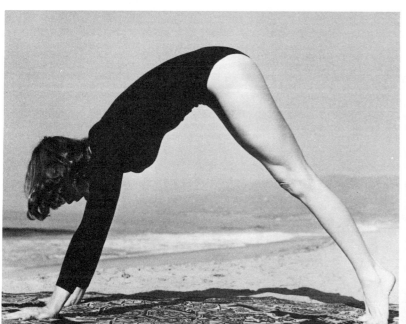

ILLUSTRATION 13.

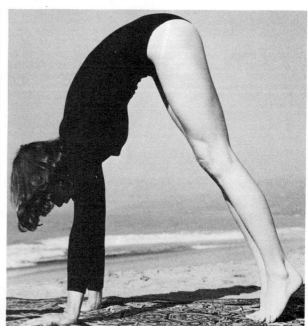

ILLUSTRATION 14.

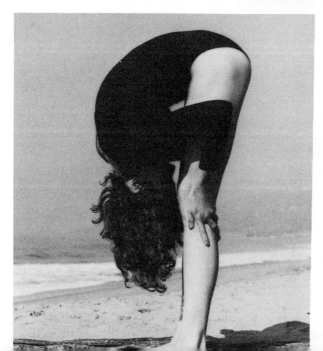

ILLUSTRATION 15.

Lower yourself to the ground onto your stomach, keeping your head raised, and reach your arms back and grab your ankles to do the Back Bend Rock. (*See illustration 16.*) You'll be surprised to find that sticking your tongue out will give your body more stretch and bend. Rock back and forth several times using your stomach muscles to do the work. You will tire after six or eight rocks if you are not in shape. Let go of your ankles and lie on your stomach, resting as long as you wish. Do a series of four rocks or six to eight rocks each time. This exercise will do wonders for your stomach but it is so powerful that you should only do it every second or third day to give your muscles a chance to strengthen themselves.

Now is a good time to rest on your back in the Fetal Position (*Pavanamuktasana*). Lifting first one leg at a time and then both, press the knees against the chest with arms crossed over the knees and raise your face so that your nose touches your knees. (*See illustration 17.*) While your knee or knees are raised, hold your breath as long as it's comfortable then exhale as you let the legs down. This is good to relieve stomach gas, to relieve constipation, and to strengthen stomach muscles.

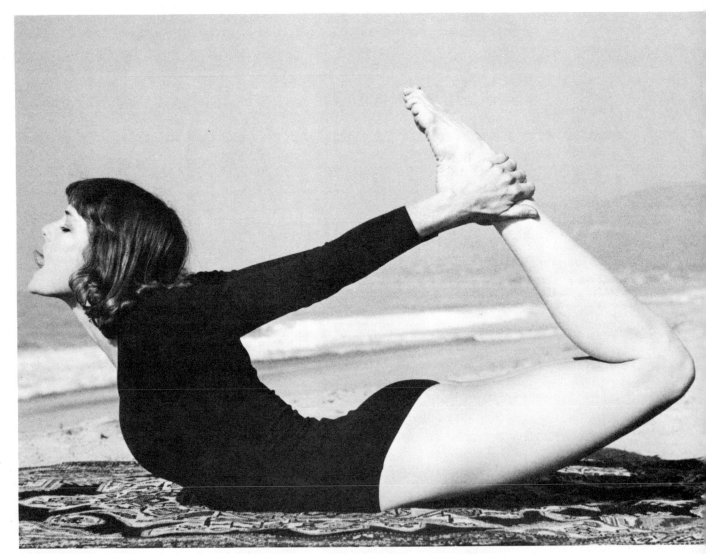

ILLUSTRATION 16.

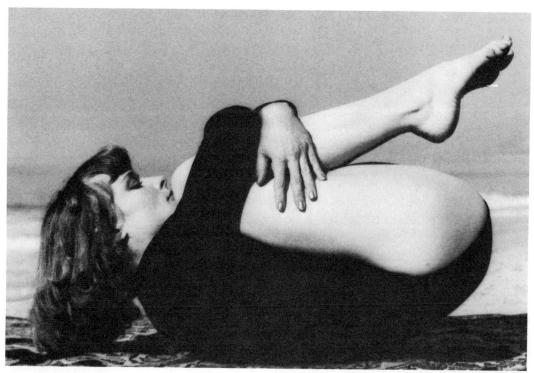

ILLUSTRATION 17.

At this point you may want to try doing a Head Stand or *Sirshasana*. It took me many years of doing simpler yoga poses to get my confidence up to even try this one, but once I decided to master it, it came easily. Some people feel that because the neck was never meant to support the weight of the body this exercise shouldn't be attempted, but there are many healthy yogis who daily prove that this isn't true. Still it *is* important to let your arms take the weight of your body rather than your neck. It's best to do the head stand near a wall just in case you lose your balance. This exercise can benefit the whole body, in particular the brain, by improving blood circulation. It is an especially good pose for meditation. Some yogis entirely eliminate all the other poses and do only *Sirshasana* for 25 to 30 minutes a day.

On bended knees with top of head resting on floor, place forearms on floor to form a triangle with locked fingers supporting back of head. Lift behind up and bring knees in close to armpits still keeping your feet on the ground. When you feel you have reached a balance point it is time to begin to lift the toes and fold the legs. When first attempting this, you may wish to stop here as this exercise should be built up gradually in stages. Once you have gained confidence, slowly fold the knees and lift the legs until the heels are touching your behind. Next continue lifting knees until they are pointing straight up and your feet form a balance parallel to the ground. Finally lift the feet up slowly until they point straight up. This position should be held only as long as comfortable—possibly a few seconds at first and building up to two or three minutes. Come down the same way—slowly. (If you must sneeze, yawn, or cough *come down first.*) A good variation on a straight-up leg position is to arch your back, letting legs go back for balance. Then come back to straight and bend forward by very gradually bringing them to a right angle with the back and finally coming down until toes touch the floor in front of you.

Next you might try the Spinal Twist (*Poorna Matsyendrasana*). Some people find this easy to do but others have considerable difficulty. It seems to depend on how limber you are when you begin. Even if you can't do it at first, keep working with it and eventually it will come to you. Sit on the floor with knees up. Lower the left knee until it touches the floor and is pointing slightly to the side, keeping the foot near the inner right thigh. Then lift the foot of the right leg over the left and place it flat on the floor next to the outside of the left knee. Now twist enough to bring the left shoulder over the outside of the right knee but bring the left arm back over the top of the right lower leg and grab the outside of the right foot. (*See illustration 18*.) All that remains is to twist the upper body a bit more toward the right and with the right arm reach around behind your back until the top of the lower arm rests flat against your back and the top of the hand extends around the left side of your waist. (*See illustration 19*.) As you do this you will probably hear several pops—this is the sound of your back straightening itself out. If you don't hear any pops right away use a twist-jerk motion a bit more to the right. If you *still* don't hear a pop you are probably already in alignment. Try to maintain this position for a full minute. Then reverse the position of your legs and arms and twist to the left. This is a good exercise to do at any time of the day when your back feels stiff or aches. At first you may want to do an easier variation where the left leg is extended straight out on the floor rather than with the knee bent. A more advanced variation which I can't do yet is to have the left leg in a Lotus position with the foot over the top of the right thigh and pressing against the abdomen. This is actually the Full Spinal Twist.

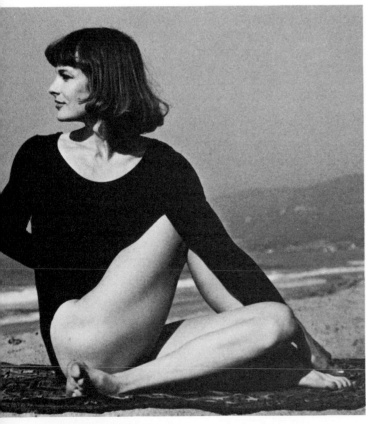

ILLUSTRATION 18.

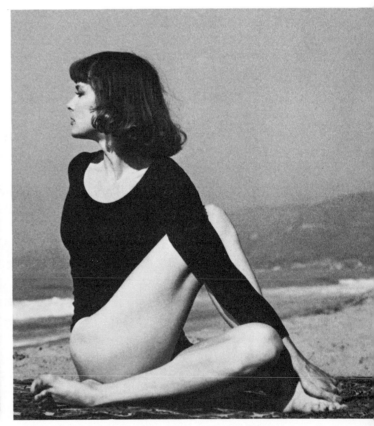

ILLUSTRATION 19.

A simple exercise you may enjoy doing is the Knee Push, a ballet warm-up. You sit with soles of feet touching and pulled in as close to the body as possible with both knees extended toward the floor. Keep your arms behind you for support. Force knees down simultaneously in a bouncing motion. Eventually you will be limber enough for the knees to touch the floor comfortably.

Another ballet exercise which follows naturally is the Stretch to Toes. Sit with both legs extended in front of you as wide apart as they will go, reach with both hands and top of head to touch pointed toes with hands and knee with head. Slowly bounce and stretch from waist with outstretched arms from left foot to center to right foot, keeping head and arms as close to the floor and stretching as much as possible.

While still sitting on floor and limbered up from stretching an easy transition is made to the Half Lotus Sandwich. The left leg is extended, the right is bent Lotus-style with the foot over the top of the left upper thigh. With the right hand reach around your back and grab the right big toe (*see illustration 20*), bend down with your head as close to the left knee as possible

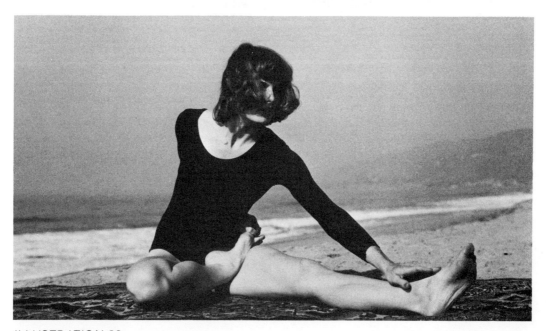

ILLUSTRATION 20.

and with the left hand grab the left toe and flex the toes while trying to get the head as close to the knee as possible. (*See illustration 21.*) Now switch and do the other leg.

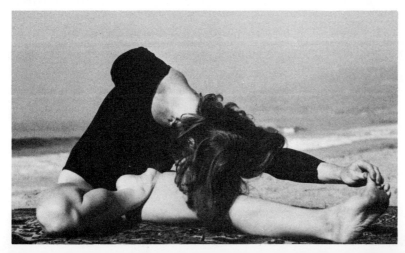

ILLUSTRATION 21.

Without moving, sit up and complete the Lotus position. Then with arms crossed in back, grab both big toes. (*See illustration 22.*) It helps to bend forward at first to reach your toes. Now reverse the position of the arms and legs. This is called the Bound Lotus (*Baddha Padmasana*) and is a good exercise for the stomach.

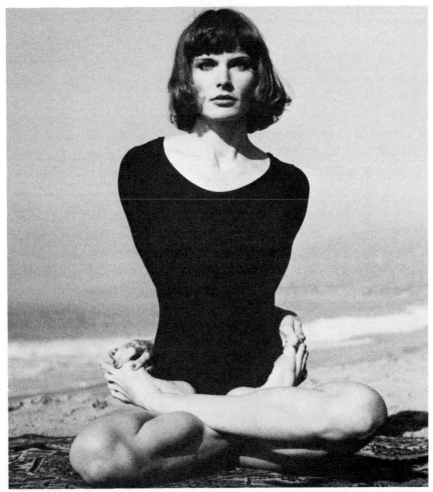

ILLUSTRATION 22.

Now let go of the toes, relax the arms by placing hands on knees in a regular Lotus and prepare to do the Stomach Rotation or *Kriya Nauli* exercise. It is very important not to strain to do this—build up your skill slowly. Take several long, smooth, deep breaths. Exhale completely and pull in all the stomach muscles until the area below the rib cage is completely concave (or sucked in). Rotate the stomach in an imaginary circle first forward, then back, then to one side in a clockwise motion, and finally to the other side in a counterclockwise motion. Inhale and repeat breathing process each time you change directions. This is great for controlling stomach flab and fat. Always do this exercise on an empty stomach, unless you are constipated in which case it is helpful to drink two cups of water or herb tea to aid elimination before starting. Yogis say this exercise restores youth and vitality to those who practice it faithfully. There are many variations on this exercise which you can learn from a book on yoga.

I like to finish up every yoga session with what I call the All Direction S-t-r-e-t-c-h. Stand with your feet about two feet apart, bend down, touch toes of right foot with both hands and lock thumbs. Slowly lean back and upward to the right allowing your hands to lead the way, stretching and leaning as far back as you can go. Very, very slowly move arms in a big circle toward the back, bending back from the waist until your arms have made a complete circle from right to left and once again you are leaning forward and touching your toes in front. Repeat this three more times and then switch to four big circles from left to right. This should take out every last little kink in your body and leave you feeling light, limber, and with an improved waistline. You can do this stretch anytime you feel a little stiff.

By the way, if you practice yoga consistently it is not even necessary to consciously change any of your poor eating and living habits because they will automatically begin to change. Eventually all ailments will begin to disappear as well. Swami Satchidananda says that after a certain point, not only is yoga a cure of all illness, but its continued practice gives permanent immunity to illness.

Aside from yoga, there are many other shortcuts you can take to keep your body in shape, some of which I imagine would fall into the category of isometrics. The way I do isometrics is not consciously thought out. I try to take the opportunity to turn every motion into a flexing and relaxing of the muscles—whether it's walking, cooking, busywork, or just standing around and talking. I usually gravitate toward something that I can use as a prop—something that resists when I push such as a table, chair, or a door jamb. Then I use the prop to lean and balance on.

I enjoy background music, especially because it is an invitation to move. Dancing is just an enlarged and more organized version of do-it-yourself isometrics. Almost any kind of movement that you can think of is good as long as it involves the effortless expansion and contraction of muscles, subtle and not so subtle. You will find that your body loves isometrics. The more you do, the better it feels. There is a whole range of things you can do from a plié to a push. I don't think you need to study isometrics if you have any imagination at all. Just experiment with movement that makes you feel good every time you get a private moment or when you feel comfortable enough to try it around a friend. It should be something that gets to be second nature to you.

If you have always been one of those people who thought that it was better to sit than to stand and to lie than to sit, now is a good time to reappraise some of your values. I understand this point of view because I used to think that it was smart to be cool, in both senses of the word. Now I look forward to the opportunity to be able to *use* my body every chance I get. It gives me energy and is mentally and physically stimulating as well as good for my figure.

On the other hand I am not trying to underestimate the value of rest. If you are one who is fortunate enough to be able to move around so much that you actually get tired and *have* to sit rather than stand, then obviously you are one person who can skip this chapter. Don't fool yourself, though, if you are always tired but never actually do anything. If you are tired from boredom or nonphysical strain, some good vigorous action, even isometrics alone, would re-energize you. By the way, waking up your body through exercise should be an adjunct to revising your eating habits to expel the tired feeling from your life entirely.

One of the best exercises of all is walking. I don't know anyone with a reasonably sound mind and body who can give me a legitimate excuse for not walking, yet I don't know many people who walk except to get from their house to their car and from their car to the building in front of which they're parked. New York City people are fortunate exceptions and probably walk more in a day than Los Angelinos walk in a week.

If you can make up for the lack of exercise by playing tennis or golf or cycling every week you are indeed lucky (and smart). But if you are one of those terribly busy and "can't be bothered to participate in sports" types, then I suggest getting out and walking. If you don't feel too silly, combine this with trotting or running. Even if you take a walk two or three times a week for an hour, it would be a big improvement over doing nothing and could be immensely physically rewarding.

Once you really get into walking for enjoyment as well as health you will start to devise walking trips to new and unusual places. You can even arrange to be dropped off and picked up while your friends ride. I think that the more you walk, the more you enjoy it. One of the best rewards is the immediate healthy glow and flushed cheeks you get when you have returned from your walk, along with a warm tingling feeling of well-being that you seldom get from doing anything else.

While I'm on the subject of exercise, there is one other prominent method of keeping the body firm and youthful and this is with massage, especially if used in combination with other types of exercise and a good diet.

It will probably be necessary to learn how to give yourself a massage. If you don't know how or if you have never had one, there are a few ways to learn. One is to get someone else to teach you by actually giving you a massage, another is getting the method explained to you, and the third is to get a good book of massage techniques.* I have learned through a combination of experiences: I've had a few professional massages, I've made a brief study of it in a few books, I've experimented a lot on myself and my friends, and I've had them help me too.

A massage is great for loosening up hardened fat deposits (sometimes referred to as cellulite). If you are melting away the pounds on a good regime to keep slim, you will probably want to "firm up" any slack skin by massage and exercise. Even when your weight is where you want it, you can continue to help keep your body in great shape by a massage about once a week, more often if you have the time. I have found that I can squeeze in two or three massages a week if I do them myself. The most convenient time for me to do it is right after my shower in the morning. I use a very light, milky foundation lotion to lubricate the skin without leaving a greasy surface. First I rub the lotion on, one limb at a time, and as I go along, I grab the skin with both hands and knead it like bread (except for the arms where you can only use one hand obviously). For the long limbs I also use a long, firm stroke along the long muscles with the tensed tips of the fingers as hard as I can take it. I give particular attention to the feet, elbows, and knees, which always need it the most.

When you are doing your own massage, don't forget the face, but use gentler, small strokes in a circular motion up and away from the center of the face, opposite gravity. Try to release the tension in areas like the forehead by massaging in the opposite direction from which lines tend to form. Around the eyes be particularly careful not to stretch the skin.

---

*Massage techniques explained and illustrated along with other exercises especially for sense awareness are contained in Getting Clear, by Anne Kent Rush. New York: Random House Inc., 1973.

Massage gently in a circular motion first in the opposite direction of natural lines and then up and out toward the hair line. Massage is also great for the skin as it improves surface circulation. I think that, aside from getting regular exercise, facial massage is one of the most important things you can do to prevent tension lines and sagging skin.

There is one other massage technique that I would like to mention here called "reflectology" which is a special kind of foot massage. Each point on the soles of the feet has a nerve ending which corresponds with a particular organ or part of the body. If you massage the bottom of the foot you can stimulate circulation and send energy through the nerves to any place in the body that needs attention. A sore spot on the foot indicates that some part is not functioning properly. There are charts available which show the sole of the foot with the corresponding organs or body parts.*

I'm not sure if using a loofah falls under massage or bathing, but no discussion of exercise in relation to health and beauty would be complete without a few words about breathing and bathing.

A loofah, if you have never seen one, looks like a large rough sponge but it is actually made from the rough, spongelike, fibrous, inner part of a large gourd. It can be used from time to time while taking a shower, bath, or sauna to lightly massage the whole body except the face and sensitive areas. It is amazing to me that the rough surface of the loofah leaves your skin so smooth that you have to feel it to believe it. This great little trick increases blood circulation immediately below the surface of the skin which not only helps the body to remove surface impurities and stimulates the growth of new cells, but also loosens and removes dead cells that clog pores and take away from a glowing skin surface. Remember, the skin, via the pores and sweat glands, is one of the major organs of elimination and must be kept clean and exercised for it to function at its best. The combination of the loofah in the shower and the massage immediately afterward will so awaken and improve your skin that you will see the visible results immediately.

When you are exercising, you should try to develop an awareness of how you breathe and maybe take some of your exercise outdoors where you will also get a refreshing blend of rich oxygen and just the right amount of nitrogen. Proper breathing should be an integral part of all your movements, in particular if you are doing yoga. In fact, the study of breathing techniques used as an adjunct to almost every pose is an integral part of Hatha (physical) yoga. The main thing to remember, whether you're doing yoga or not, is to breathe through your nostrils (rather than from your mouth), letting the diaphragm pull in the air and then push it out. This encourages deep breathing from the lowest point that air can reach in your body before letting it out into the atmosphere. There are many other techniques for breathing that improve circulation and other specific bodily functions which can be learned from a study of Hatha yoga.

*Stories the Feet Can Tell, by Eunice D. Ingham. P.O. Box 948, Rochester, New York; also in Getting Clear by Anne Kent Rush.

CHAPTER SIX

SKIN, HAIR, AND MAKEUP

Skin

Diet is the single most important consideration in seeking beautiful skin, as you have already learned, but there are lots of things that you can do to your skin's exterior that will aid in keeping it beautiful.

Exercise not only keeps your body healthy but your skin as well. Masks and massages can achieve the same results for your face as walking or yoga or dance do for your body, by increasing the circulation of your blood.

A good mask, when it is still drying, has the property of drawing blood close to the skin's surface where it can draw out toxins and other impurities. Then when it is rinsed off, the blood shoots to the surface, increasing stimulation to the skin.

A fine quality clay or organic volcanic ash is one of the best masks for oily skin although there are many good commercial ones too. Potions Eternal puts out a mint-flavored, ginseng, vitamin E clay mask. Cattier of France distributes a fine green clay and also a mask made from almond, olive oil, and the same fine green clay (the oil is added to this mask because the clay is so drying that even for oily skin a slightly softer texture is more pleasant). For both cleansing and drying overoily skin, partly beaten egg whites alone have made a good mask for such famous beauties as Marie Antoinette and one of Goya's models, the Duchess of Alba.

Another famous beauty had a different recipe for keeping skin beautiful. She would boil a combination of milk, lemon juice, and brandy and apply it warm to the skin twice a day for as long as she lived. An equally effective method I think would be to gently heat one-eighth of a cup of milk mixed with the juice of half a lemon, splash on the face, let dry for a few minutes, and then rinse and gently pat dry.

Astringents like lemon juice, apple cider vinegar or blended strawberries are sometimes used in oily skin masks. These can be used individually as an astringent face lotion but should be diluted with water first.

Other binders besides clay and egg whites are yogurt, buttermilk, oatmeal, yeast cake paste, or almond meal.

The very drying atmosphere of artificially cooled or heated environments, exposure to toxins in the air especially concentrated in cities and downtown areas where there is a lot of traffic, overexposure to the harsh elements of sun and wind, the constant use of makeup which causes wear and tear just in application and removal, and the increasingly devitalized diets of today's average American all contribute to problems of dry skin.

Please don't misinterpret what I am saying by going overboard with moisturizers. Even a very dry skin will benefit more from a light moisturizer than from a heavy, oily one. And it should be sparingly applied according to how much the skin absorbs without looking oily. For me, it is usually enough to rub the moisturizer all over my hands as though I were using hand lotion, and then to gently pat only the areas of my face that need it the most. One more light application on my hands covers my neck, which is even dryer than my face.

Some masks act specifically as moisturizers although all masks do this to some extent. The mere fact that a mask prevents evaporation of the skin's surface moisture means that when you remove it the skin has an accumulation of moisture that you couldn't get in any more efficient way. Theoretically Vaseline is the best moisturizer (according to David Anderson, Director and Vice President of Max Factor's research and development department) for the same reason although no one I know finds wearing Vaseline a pleasant experience. Natural moisturizing masks usually include natural vegetable oil like avocado, safflower, peanut, corn, olive, wheat germ, vitamins E and A, or almond oil; mashed or blended fruits or vegetables chosen for their moisturizing effect and for their soothing and healing qualities; and honey, egg yolk, sour cream, or mashed banana as a binder. Buttermilk soaked in cotton and dabbed on the face makes a good lotion after a cleansing or can be used as a binder in a mask for either oily or dry skin. Glycerin is also commonly added to masks or moisturizing lotions for its particularly good natural moisturizing ability. Glycerin is made from vegetable sources and can be purchased at a drugstore.

Tapping the fingers gently in honey and applying it to the face provides excellent stimulation and tone to the skin as well as being an excellent natural moisturizer. This technique has been used by Louise Long and her followers in giving facials to such stars as Garbo, Deitrich, Kim Novak, and many others over the years.

Under a mask the skin supposedly has the increased ability to absorb nutrients from the food you put on it although cosmetic manufacturers maintain that there is nothing that you can put on your skin, with the exception of one or two highly potent and dangerous drugs, that will penetrate any more than the surface level. Cosmetics manufactured in this country are not allowed to contain any drugs which penetrate the skin for fear that the skin will be susceptible to absorbing poisons in the atmosphere or anywhere near the person wearing this type of cosmetic.

On consulting with David Anderson, of Max Factor, I learned that there is no way for vitamins or specially prepared skin nutrients to actually be absorbed into the subcutaneous layers of the skin. Surface penetration goes no deeper than the outermost part of the epidermis which, as in the case of a moisturizer, only tends to soften the dead or weather-worn skin of the very top layer.

This point of view was confirmed by Doree South, an "esthetician" or skin beauty expert trained in Europe. She, however, has a galvanic current machine imported from Europe that sends a low voltage electrical vibration through the specific part of the body that is being worked on enabling the second and third layers of the skin to absorb nutrients which have been applied to the surface in the form of a nutrient-moisturizer.*

On the other hand I have had people tell me, and have read in books, that because the skin both breathes and eliminates, it also has the ability to absorb what you put on its surface. This seems logical to me, too, but as yet no one has been able to prove that it is possible for this to happen.

In the meantime I see no reason to avoid nutrient preparations, except the prohibitively expensive ones and use the less expensive organic ones straight from your refrigerator. I continue to use vitamin E oil straight from the capsule to protect and nourish my lips, to heal scars or burns, and to protect the sensitive skin around my eyes.

Aside from masks, there is very little you can actually do to add moisture to the skin to any depth although I find moisturizers indispensable in beauty treatments because they protect and soften the outermost layer. The best moisturizers contain water to plump up the dehydrated skin's surface and a small amount of oil to keep the water from evaporating.

If you have dry skin, a moisturizer used sparingly should protect it at all times. But remember, too much oil can drag down the skin, reducing its elasticity and its ability to breathe. Moisturizer should only be applied in the specific spots where it is needed and these spots vary with every face. Normally the dry spots are the cheeks, jaws, and neck (which should always be considered as part of the face).

Some beauty experts, including the late Erno Lazlo, are against applying moisturizers containing oil of any kind as the skin doesn't actually absorb the oil. He claimed that skin subjected to continuous applications of oil will adjust to this unnatural condition and cease to supply its own natural oils. Although in principle this makes a lot of sense, in practice it fails to take into account the rather important consideration of environmental conditions, in particular when dealing with normal to dry skins.

I gave the Lazlo method a good, long trial period several years ago and ended up consulting a dermatologist because not only was my skin cracking and scaling, but it was breaking out with tiny little pimples that looked like a rash. The first thing the doctor said was something about the unusually dehydrated condition of my skin. It was to this that he attributed the breaking out. Evidently, this treatment just wasn't right for *my* skin.

As if once wasn't enough, fairly recently I was persuaded to try this method again, time having faded my memory somewhat. Once again, I had the same unpleasant experience, but this time I stopped before my skin had a chance to become really dry. So I went back to my old time-tried method of using a light, milky moisturizer (DuBarry Hypo-allergenic Foundation Lotion) recommended to me when I first started modeling by Beverly Damon, who had the most beautiful, young skin I have ever seen on anyone over thirty.

In a pinch I always use milk right from the refrigerator dabbed on with cotton pads, and when my eyes are tired or burning from the smog I lie down with milk-soaked cotton pads

---

*Doree also works with other highly advanced equipment such as a vaporisator to open pores and with ozone to supply oxygen to blood cells, a vacuum to prepare the skin to remove surface impurities, and a Firmator Liniette machine with goat hair bristles for brushing and removing dead tissues. Doree has just recently obtained a Depilatron, a special new machine which is a permanent hair remover to take the place of electrolysis. It works on a radio-frequency current with no needles inserted and is absolutely painless. For additional information *contact* Doree South, 409 N. Robertson, Beverly Hills, Calif. 90048.

over my eyes for a few minutes to refresh them and plump up the skin around them. This is a quick pickup to use before an evening out. As a matter of fact mayonnaise (especially the homemade type), yogurt, sour cream, or buttermilk all make good cleanser-moisturizers.

Heavy or sticky night creams and oils should be avoided as they *do* drag down the skin and stretch delicate skin around the eyes if the application is done with a heavy hand. However, a light oil like vitamin E from the capsule or avocado or olive oil lightly and sparingly patted into the skin around the eyes after cleansing the face offers good protection and lubrication, probably enough to last until the next time you wash your face.

Since no two skins are alike there are no firm rules as to how much and what kinds of moisturizing and lubricating preparations you should use. Let your skin tell you: If it is shiny and oily, then you probably either use too much or too heavy a moisturizer, or you don't need a moisturizer at all. You may require a toner or astringent lotion and more frequent washings instead. If it is a little rough, dry, or scaly, then you need to apply moisturizer more often but not necessarily one which is oilier.

The only times I can think of that an oily moisturizer should be used are when you are swimming and sunning, skiing, driving in an open-air sports car, or otherwise getting harsher than normal exposure to the elements. Another exception would be to use oil as a temporary mask to build up the skin's moisture although I don't recommend this on oily skin. If your skin is especially rough and dry, clean your face first and then lie down and apply pads of cotton soaked in hot oil (but not *too* hot) all over your face and leave them there while you rest for twenty minutes or so. Any kind of vegetable oil heated in a double boiler is fine (I prefer the smell of almond oil). The oil with the least amount of smell is safflower oil. I also smear on tahini (ground sesame seed in its own natural oil) and lie down for a few minutes while it soaks into my skin and then rinse it off in the shower.

If my skin seems especially dry, when I am in the shower or taking a hot bath I apply a liquid oil to my face immediately after washing it and leave it on until I am through bathing. The heavy steam opens up the pores and allows the oils to lubricate much deeper than when closed and dry, and the nonporous film of the oil builds up the skin's natural moisture beneath it in a kind of reserve.

I find that this is also the perfect time to give myself a facial massage because my skin is lubricated well enough for the balls of my fingers to move lightly over the skin. Relaxed and radiant is the way I feel after having imaginatively massaged each muscle.

To remove the excess oil, it usually suffices to rinse my face seconds before de-tubbing and then to pat it dry. But you should check your skin after a few minutes and if there are any remaining dry spots, sparingly pat on a bit of milky moisturizer. If there are any oily spots, they can be absorbed with special oil-drinking papers like Face Savers or facial tissues.

Another one of my favorite shower tricks which has become a weekly routine for me is to use a facial scrub consisting of kelp, sea salt, honey, comfrey, rose hips, and ginseng. This is the concoction of Rachel Perry's Potions Eternal line called "Mother Neptune's Sea Pack."* Its function is to draw out impurities, remove dead skin, and pep up skin tone. Your skin is

*Have your favorite health food store or boutique order this product from: Potions Eternal, 8441 Ridpath Dr., Los Angeles, Ca. 90046. Some of the other products I like are the Atlantis Skin Drink (moisturizer), Slumber Skin Food #1 (Vitamin E creme for eyes at night), Bathsheba's Bodily Pleasures (body lotion), Waves of the Nile (pH shampoo), and Salome's Unveiling (the clay mask I mentioned earlier). Ask for a list of other products too.

most receptive to this scrub when you apply it to a hot, wet face after having washed it, with your hands hot and wet as well. Even though my skin is slightly on the dry side, it never leaves my skin feeling too dry. If your skin is oilier you might want to leave it on for a few minutes, but I don't usually leave it on long. *I* have never tried to make it, but if this product is not available, it wouldn't be too hard to put together something that would work for you. I find that using this scrub helps prevent skin eruptions and I feel that it would be very good for someone who is trying to clear up a badly broken-out face. Helena Rubenstein Beauty Washing grains are good for normal skin and can be bought in most drugstores.

As I mentioned earlier, using a loofah on the less sensitive areas of your skin will also remove dead skin and impurities and improve your skin tone.

An effective body scrub consists of milk- or water-diluted cornmeal either with or without the loofah. By the way, one tablespoon of cornmeal can also be occasionally added to facials for removing surface impurities.

As another body scrub, you may also want to try the more complicated method of applying warmed vegetable oil to your body while standing in the tub and then, being careful to avoid the eyes and sensitive areas, rub on granular kelp with a loofah or a washcloth.* Sea salt or ordinary table salt rubbed over the less sensitive areas of the body does essentially the same thing for oiler skins.

When I get out of the shower I put the tiniest bit of moisturizer on my face and, if I have the time, I give my body a complete rubdown/massage with the aid of a lubricating body lotion. Here again I am happy to recommend another pH-balanced Potions Eternal product called "Bathsheba's Bodily Pleasures" which comes in many almost eatable flavors and is made strictly from pure, natural organic oils and vitamins.

If your body's skin is oily and broken out you may want to do your massage with lotion before your shower although you should really give more attention to correcting your diet than toning your skin at this point.

If you have oily skin, as an after-shower lotion you may prefer to rub a piece of peeled cucumber over the body. This will leave your skin especially refreshed in the summer as well as imparting a natural acid mantle. If you have a sunburn this is great therapy for any kind of skin.

Assuming that you are a woman (although I hope that many men will read and benefit from this book too), you probably wear a small amount of makeup during the day and perhaps more at night. No matter what you may have read about makeup being good for your face, even though it is now better than ever, the best possible situation for your skin is no foundation at all and either toner or moisturizer (depending on whether your skin is oily or dry) to protect your skin from today's smog. Even though I *never* cover my face with a foundation makeup unless it is required by my work, I usually wear a blusher gel or creme rouge to highlight my cheekbones, and touch up discolorations and blemishes with pan stick (a thick, oily based makeup in a tube) lightly brushed on only where needed and then set it with powder. I also wear eye makeup most of the time and sometimes lipstick. So you see, even for me, it is important to have a good cleansing program, and if you insist on wearing a foundation (overall skin coverage), it is even more important. Your skin should at least have a

Organic Make-up, by Dian Buchman. New York: Ace Books, 1975.

chance to breathe and revitalize itself at night when you are sleeping, so this cleansing is most appropriate before going to bed.

Makeup should be removed as gently as possible so as not to stretch and irritate the skin. I find that a light vegetable oil or a liquid cleanser is best and I particularly like oily pads made expressly for removing eye makeup. With a kleenex I gently blot off all the excess oil, especially around the eyes and then wash my face.

If you are not familiar with the term *pH balanced,* now would be a good time to explain it. As you already know, the body's interior, in particular the bloodstream, must always be maintained at a slightly alkaline level. But the body's exterior, the skin, will always adjust itself to having a slightly acid covering, or mantle as it is sometimes called, to give it protection from the elements. Some people have an over-acid-producing skin which makes their skin dry and sensitive. Others have skin which produces too much alkalinity making their skin too oily. If your face becomes shiny during the day, it is oily even if it feels dry. No matter what you put on your skin the body will strive to neutralize alkalinity and produce its own acid mantle. My first question when I heard this was "Then why is it so important to use products that are pH balanced to leave your skin with an acid mantle when your skin does it anyway?" The answer is that it *isn't* terribly important, but alkaline products, used over long periods of time, subject your skin to slightly harsher than necessary wear and tear. So if you want to save your skin the work, use products that are pH balanced, which means that they are more acid than alkaline.

Mary Crenshaw, in her book *The Natural Way to Super Beauty,* recommends testing all your cosmetics and beauty preparations with nitrazine or pHenaphthazine papers in the 4.5 (nature's balance) to 7.5 range. If they turn the paper purple indicating alkalinity (which happens around 5.5), then she says the product shouldn't be used. This I think is a bit extreme sice 99 out of 100 products on the market today are above the 5.5 range but are still not terribly alkaline. I only know of two lines of beauty preparations made in this country whose products are completely pH balanced: Potions Eternal and Redken. Erno Lazlo also has mostly pH-balanced products. The Pier Auge line from France can also be purchased at better department stores in this country.

Some experts feel that a regular nondetergent soap like Ivory, or an olive-oil based Castile soap or one of the super-fatted soaps should be used for washing the face because even though it has an alkaline pH, it is the most effective method to cut the grease and remove deep skin impurities. But if you have very sensitive skin like me and you don't wear much makeup, then you may prefer to use a pH-balanced soap like the one that Redken makes. I reserve the regular soaps for when I have a *real* cleaning job like after a TV show where my face and body have been covered with heavy makeup.

When washing my face I start out with soap and tepid water using only my hands so that surface impurities are washed away before the pores completely open up; then I make the water quite hot to finish the rinsing. The hot water stimulates circulation, relaxes facial muscles, and stimulates the skin to release its own oils. This is also a perfect time to use a facial scrub if you wish. It used to be considered de rigueur to finish washing the face with a cold water splash to close the pores, but I don't think this is necessary as long as you don't run right out into the smog or put on makeup immediately. In fact, I sometimes like to leave the pores open so that my skin is more receptive to the small amount of moisturizer which I pat on afterward. Still, a cold-water splash is great to stimulate circulation.

If your skin is oily, or as an occasional break from moisturizers, you may prefer to use a pH-balanced toner or tonic to close the pores or a little cold water mixed with fresh lemon juice which also leaves your skin properly pH balanced. Cold water, however, or ice packs (but don't overdo it) can be used to reduce redness in your face after you have just had a vigorous facial.

Every once in awhile if my skin seems clogged up or broken out, I give myself an herb-steam treatment which feels so great that I'm sure it helps psychologically as much as it actually helps in pushing out impurities. I use two heaping tablespoons of camomile flower tops in about a quart of boiling spring or distilled water. Any other herb teas you have on hand will work, and the herbal laxative "Swiss Kriss" (the invention of Gaylord Hauser) does the same thing. When this tea has simmered for a minute or two, remove it from the heat and put it on a low table where you can sit with your face over it, with a towel over your head and the pot, making a tentlike enclosure to keep the steam concentrated on your face. Move your face around to let the steam penetrate every pore of your skin and stay as close to the steam as you can bear. Five to ten minutes later when your face is dripping from sweat and steam and the heat is no longer strong, you are through. (Additional sweat can be induced by adding oil or honey to the face before steaming.) You can close the pores with a toner or any of the other methods I've suggested, but be sure your hands are clean as this is the time when your face is the most susceptible to impurities and harmful bacteria.

I have had facials done by experts only a few times in my life and they all tell you the same thing. Don't ever pick at or squeeze your pimples or blackheads. Let the expert armed with a magnifying glass approach you from the right angle to do it or don't do it at all. For myself I say "nonsense," because I have learned through experience to know when a blackhead or pimple is ready to be gently squeezed out. I have, however, several fingernail scars from trying to take out a pimple that was either too deep or not ready to come. It is for this very reason that the experts say hands off, and as a general rule "hands off" *is* best.

Up to this point I have only considered normal skin and its oily or dry variations. But having been a teenager with embarrassing acne, I feel obliged to mention special treatments for this condition.

Acne is a result of overactivity in the production of oils released by the sebaceous glands. It is a logical guess that this gland is easily set off kilter by suppressed or unexpressed emotional problems. At the time that it was happening to me, I wasn't aware that I had emotional problems but now that I think about it I was on the brink of breaking away from my family and probably had many anxieties and rebellious ideas that needed release. But there was no help in the offing, especially from my family. How could they possibly understand all that I was feeling? If this ever happens to you, it wouldn't be a bad idea to get a go-between of some sort to hear you out and give you some good advice to benefit you as well as your family for the time being.

Improving your diet (which is usually pretty bad when you are feeling bad yourself) will help you to come out of a mental slump faster than you expect because it starts improving your skin so rapidly that you start wanting to go out and show your face to the world again.

If you have been subsisting on the typical teenage-American diet of burgers, chocolate shakes, fries, cokes, and candy bars then be prepared to do an about-face or keep the one you've got. A good diet for an over-oily skin is basically the same one I have talked about throughout this book, although there are a few points that should be stressed.

Fried foods and hydrogenated fats are the hardest ones to get out of your system and look the worst—poised like a volcano ready to erupt under your skin. Cold-pressed vegetable oil in moderate amounts (at least two tablespoons a day) helps loosen up and expel hardened fats. A little granular lecithin sprinkled on cereal, desserts, and salads will accomplish the same thing, but use this in addition to the oil. It is a good idea to cut out almost all animal fats including foods like whole milk, cheese, butter, fatty meats, and whole eggs for the time being. (An exception would be poached eggs with most of the white cut off, eaten for breakfast with a bit of bran sprinkled on.) These can gradually be added back to the diet in small amounts when the skin improves. Fish is a good choice for protein as it contains a relatively small amount of fat. Skim milk is another good source of protein. Raw egg yolks in a "smoothie" are fine too.

Try to have at least two meals a day that include raw vegetables and cooked vegetables, preferably the green leafy type, to assist in elimination of toxins and for vitamin A. Acne is indicative of a clogged system which requires a lot of roughage to loosen up and eliminate obstructions.

I have heard that chocolate stays in the system two weeks before it can be eliminated; rather constipating wouldn't you say? Other constipating foods are refined breads, potatoes, grains, sugar, and junk or snack foods, and are best eliminated entirely unless you can find the same things made with unrefined products. Even then, the amounts should be cut to minimal proportions. Cheese and nuts are also constipating and should be taken in moderation. I hope I don't have to remind you that soft drinks, sugar, and other refined sweets should be avoided and desserts made with honey should be minimized for the time being. Fresh juicy fruits (except pineapple) between meals or fruit as a meal in itself will also be a great aid in cleansing the toxins from your system if consumed in moderate amounts. Fresh-juiced vegetable cocktails of combinations like carrots, cucumber, romaine, and alfalfa sprouts are great between meals to clear up the skin.

As I mentioned earlier, when I took steps to clear up a suddenly *bad* acne condition, the combination of this diet with an injection of antibiotics to combat the infections, and vitamin A to make up for all the greens I wasn't getting, caused an immediate, visible reversal in the condition of my skin. Within a week I was well on my way to my naturally clear skin after having put up with the embarrassment of increasingly bad acne for almost a year. A rather spectacular recovery! My only regret was that I could have saved myself a lot of agony by seeing a dermatologist a lot sooner than I did!

The hardest part of regaining my clear skin was the rule of NO MAKEUP! Because ruptured, puffy skin is nothing you want anyone to see, I was wearing thick gooey makeup (supposedly medicated) to cover it up but this only aggravated the condition and caused more infections. All the doctor allowed me to wear was calamine lotion, which is very drying and contains absolutely no oil. Today there are water-based hypo-allergenic makeups on the market which would be a good substitute. I was instructed to wash my face with a good antibacterial soap and water as hot as I could bear three times a day in order to facilitate a drying and peeling process that would remove the top layer or two of skin which included of course, the most part of my fast-disappearing acne. (Soaps containing chemicals are harmful when used over a long period of time.) If your skin ever feels as though it's getting too dry, cut down on the washings. Now, I would also use a mask regularly.

For a mask, the old-time procedure of rubbing a raw, peeled tomato or potato on your face is a good, mild remedy for blemishes. But if you wish to try something with more "drawing" power, plain clay (the type I mentioned earlier) or a yeast cake moistened with water is one of the most simple and effective methods you can find. If you want to try something special, moisten a little clay, oatmeal, and cornmeal with milk, add enough egg white to make it good and sticky, and after massaging it into the skin where needed, allow it to dry at least twenty minutes before rinsing. Or, to save some mixing time, use oatmeal moistened with milk and/or yogurt. This becomes a scrub instead of a facial if you massage it gently into your skin.

I was told absolutely to keep my hands off my face and never to squeeze a pimple. I would add to this washing your hair every day or two so that its natural oils won't aggravate the skin. At the time, I was living in Hawaii and getting a lot of sun. I was happy to hear that a small amount of sun every day would actually help my skin to get better faster. Fifteen minutes is fine.

Recipes for Facials, Masks, Baths, and Drinks

Avocado Facial

To moisturize the skin, mash a couple teaspoons of avocado and half a teaspoon of lemon juice together and apply to face and neck for about twenty minutes. Then rinse.

Antiblemish Potato Rub

Just as the title says, rub a raw, peeled piece of potato over your face to help clear up blemishes. You can also peel and grate a raw potato, spread it over your face while you are lying down for twenty minutes, and then rinse.

Skin-Feeding Facial

To retard wrinkles and lines around the eyes, feed your skin a capsule of vitamin E or wheat germ oil blended with an egg yolk and 1 teaspoon of honey. Leave on your face for twenty minutes before rinsing.

Carrot Juice Facial

This is good for general toning and moisturizing: Blend together two teaspoons carrot juice, either an egg white if you have oily skin or an egg yolk if you have dry skin, one tablespoon honey, and one teaspoon lecithin dissolved in the carrot juice (this is optional to add a finer texture to the skin). Apply this mixture to your face, leave for twenty minutes and then rinse.

Papaya Facial

To help increase circulation on the surface of the skin, mash two or three tablespoons papaya and blend with one tablespoon sour cream and one tablespoon honey. Smooth on face gently and leave for twenty minutes before rinsing.

Eucalyptus Oil Bath

Add a few drops of eucalyptus oil to your bath for a refreshing, heavenly smelling experience.

Yeast Mask

Add enough water to soften brewer's yeast flakes (or one cake of yeast for more drawing and drying power) and make it into a paste. Oil the skin first and then apply the mask for fifteen or twenty minutes. This is particularly good for blackheads and oily skin, although dry skin can benefit from its tightening effect once or twice a month. Yeast paste can also be added to other facial recipes like the ones suggested in this book for additional tightening.

Oatmeal Facial

This will moisturize dry skin: Mix together one beaten egg yolk, one tablespoon cooked oatmeal, one tablespoon honey, and a few drops of lemon juice. Apply this to the face for twenty minutes and then rinse.

A Great Drink to Clear Up the Skin From Inside

In between meals or as a meal substitute, juice one cucumber or one bunch of green string beans in your juicer; then juice one or two of the following: one or two carrots, one small bunch of parsley, one small bunch of watercress, one small bunch of alfalfa sprouts, two cups torn spinach, or two cups torn beet tops. Combine juices and drink immediately. This formula can be varied according to your taste and what vegetables you happen to have in your refrigerator.

Banana Facial

To tighten and moisturize the skin, mash about one-third of a banana until it is smooth, blend in one teaspoon honey and apply to your face for twenty minutes before rinsing off.

Healing Milk Facial

To heal blemishes and soothe chapped skin use one tablespoon milk, one tablespoon honey, and a beaten egg yolk for dry skin or a beaten egg white for oily skin. Apply it to your face for twenty minutes and then rinse.

Gelatin Mask

To moisturize and soften the skin, dissolve one tablespoon gelatin with a little boiling water, add a few drops of lemon juice, and one tablespoon honey. Apply the resulting mixture to a clean face, leave for twenty minutes, and then rinse.

If you feel an astringent is helpful to close the pores after your facial or at any other time, equal parts of either lemon juice or apple-cider vinegar and water are easy to mix and store in the refrigerator for a few days at a time.

How to Smell Sweet From Inside

Toxins and poorly digested foods cause bad body odors and bad breath respectively. Eating a diet with lots of highly alkaline vegetables will help to eliminate toxins and neutralize acids, PLUS, if the vegetables are very green you have the added advantage of chlorophyll which is a natural deodorizer. Have juiced greens occasionally in place of a meal, eat lots of steamed or raw greens with your meals, or take an occasional daily fast consisting of only soup made from greens like this one:

Bieler Broth
To 2 quarts of boiling water or vegetable broth add:
2 cups chopped celery
2 cups chopped green beans
season with herbs, kelp, and paprika
Boil covered for 3 minutes and add:
2 cups chopped zucchini
2 cups chopped parsley

Reduce flame to medium and cook 5 minutes more. Then put whole mixture through blender and serve with a pat of butter, a sprinkling of paprika and a glop of yogurt if you wish. This should last one day for two people. For a different texture, hold aside ¼ to ½ the mixture before blending and add back to soup after blending.

This regime won't work too well unless you are improving your diet in general and have already begun to eliminate an excess of highly toxic, indigestible, and acid foods and improper combinations.

Dr. Bieler calls live yeast the poor man's sodium-rich vegetable; it can be taken on an empty stomach occasionally to do the same thing as the green vegetables.

Hair

Healthy hair, just like your skin and other parts of your body, is beautiful only because it is well-nourished from the inside and well-groomed on the outside. If your system is in prime condition because you eat intelligently and if you treat your hair with respect, the inevitable result is shiny, lively hair with vibrant color.

I think I have seen my hair go through every possible change—from complete disaster to absolutely beautiful, which is the way it is now.

The worst disasters came from bleaching it, or overbleaching it, I should say. And I have known at least two ladies who got overpermed because they were already overbleached and ended up with a real disaster—no hair!

And then there are all the other stages in between which can be avoided by learning a few basic things. I hope hairdressers don't hate me, but the more you learn to do for yourself at home (or at least have an understanding of) the better off your hair will be. This is not to say that your hairdresser isn't competent, because most of them are; it is just that no one can get to know your hair better than you and YOU should know it very well! For beginners, keeping it clean and frequently cut disposes your hair to its best behavior so you can get to know its better side.

Getting your hair to hang naturally may take some practice, at least it did for me. This was due mainly to the fact that I had never let it dry properly. That's right. I never got out of the shower, blotted my hair dry, tossed it about to loosen it up, and let it dry naturally. My hair had always been straight but I noticed that in very humid weather, tiny curls would form around my hairline when my hair was pulled back in a band. I vaguely realized that my hair must have some curl in it but never thought of or knew how to bring it out. I had long hair for years and when I was finally ready for a change, off it came. The English-schoolboy cut didn't work because it turned out that there was quite a bit of curl in my hair. I had reached a point where I wanted my hair to be completely natural: no fussing, no setting, no dryers. It was hard to get used to the fact that I have semicurly hair as I had always thought of myself as having straight hair.

To complicate matters even further I had had my hair cut in Paris and was vacationing on the island of Sardinia when I discovered my curls. Who could be bothered with straightening hair to comform to an English-schoolboy cut there? I desperately wanted another haircut, but there were no competent hairdressers around. So one day I got out some scissors and decided to attempt it myself. I only dared because I was already pretty good at cutting hair for some of my friends and relatives. But on myself it was suddenly a different story. I was totally undecided about how I wanted it to look, so starting that day I began the long process of gradually cutting my hair, a little at a time, until one day it finally looked perfect. I have been changing it since then to suit whatever I am doing, but I'm no longer timid about giving myself a haircut.

That period of liberation was great, but I could never be satisfied with one style forever. My hair is longer now, but this time with a more dramatic cut that looks great either dried naturally or set in any way that appeals to me at the moment. This is the most versatile my hair has ever been and it is due to being free and able to style and cut it whenever it seems right for me to change.

You don't have to be able to cut hair to have this freedom, although it helps. If you can decide on a definite style and find a hairdresser with whom you can work in a positive direction, then stick with him and always communicate to him exactly what you want.

To do your own hair styling and cutting, I suggest you try to figure out how the hair of someone whose hairstyle you like was cut or you can do this by going through some fashion magazines.

For those of you who are brave, I am devoting some space to the actual cutting of hair which is the real nitty gritty of getting hair that falls perfectly no matter what you do to it.

My favorite current haircut is one that allows the hair to be blown and tossed about a bit without falling into the eyes. It can be either short or long. It lies beautifully because it is cut in a curve around the face and in a curve from top to bottom. It is called the "all one length" haircut when it is about two inches long, but there are many variations for longer styles which I like even better.

Before you start a haircut you, of course, need scissors, the kind made for blunt cutting with a three-and-one-quarter-inch cutting blade; and a hard rubber rat-tail comb with medium teeth (Champion makes a good one available at local beauty supply stores).

I start with the hair completely wet, carefully brushed or combed out, parted in the middle and combed straight down and slightly toward the front. Then I comb the bangs into my noncutting hand and hold the comb while I cut, just below my fingers, switching the scissors to the hand holding the hair as I comb.

If there is to be a fringe (bangs), I measure about one inch lower than the eyebrows and cut an upside-down V right out of the middle. Then gently curving away from the upside-down V, I cut down the sides of the hair, alternating my cutting from one side to the other as the hair is cut longer and longer until it curves all around to the back and joins the other side in the middle. Add an inch to the length you think it should be because when it dries it gets back the bounce it loses when it's wet. And even longer "allowance for bounce" is needed for *very* curly hair. Some of the extra length is also an allowance for some of the hair which will be cut even shorter in the next step and then will need trimming again. If you are wearing your hair straight or in a page boy with an absolutely blunt cut, here is where the hair cut ends. In this case you don't need to allow for more than a half inch for "bounce." By the way, this style of hair cut often looks great with the bangs cut straight across (see *illustration 1*). An even more dramatic version of this cut follows the brow line all the way to the ear and the rest of the hair is cut shoulder length (see *illustration 2*).

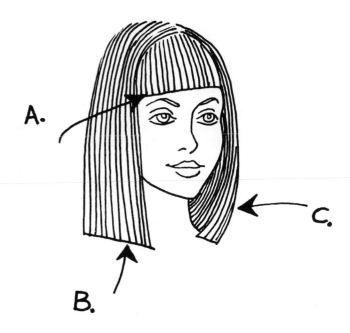

A.

B.

C.

ILLUSTRATION 1. FOR A BLUNT CUT, JUST SCISSOR ABSOLUTELY STRAIGHT ACROSS THE BANGS ABOUT A HALF-INCH OVER THE EYEBROWS (ARROW A) AND STRAIGHT ACROSS THE BOTTOM (ARROW B). USING A BRUSH AND A BLOW DRYER, YOU CAN TURN THE ENDS UNDER (ARROW C).

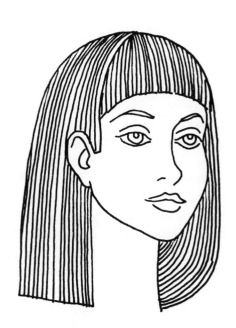

ILLUSTRATION 2. THIS IS ANOTHER BLUNT CUT, WITH THE BANGS GOING ALL THE WAY TO THE EARS. HERE, TOO, A BLOW DRYER SHAPES THE HAIR NICELY.

The next step is what I call back cutting. With the tail of your rat-tail comb, you measure a section of hair about a half inch thick and two inches long, comb it straight out away from the head. Just past where your fingers hold it, cut it at an angle up toward the top of the head so that each hair falls shorter than the one below it—like the branches of a Christmas tree. (See *illustration 3.*)

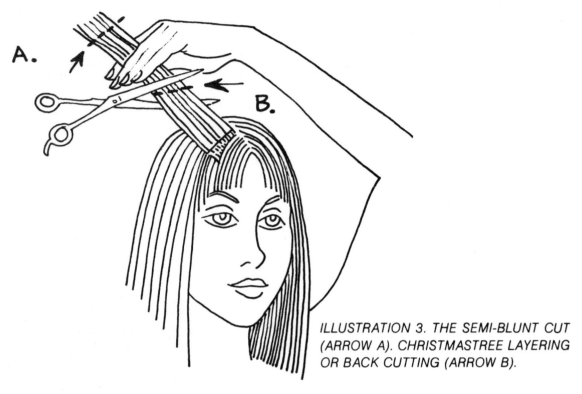

ILLUSTRATION 3. THE SEMI-BLUNT CUT (ARROW A). CHRISTMASTREE LAYERING OR BACK CUTTING (ARROW B).

Going all around the head you hold out these thin vertical sections of hair, adding a few of the adjacent hairs which you have just cut, and you have a guide to measure how long the next one should be. As you go from front to back, the hair will be cut progressively longer and longer using the length of the bangs and the gradually lengthening sides as a guide.

If you want a shagged effect, you can back cut it, cutting up *into the hair,* imitating an exaggerated Christmas tree effect. Or you can cut it in a modified curve parallel to the scalp, slightly rounded at either end for a longer, more blunt-cut look. While working on this part, shake the head around and loosen the hair with your fingers to see how it is falling. If the hair looks thick in one spot it is probably because it needs more back cutting.

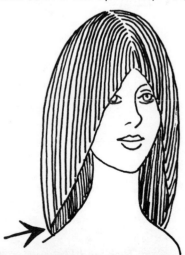

EVEN FOR A LAYERED LOOK, YOU START WITH A BLUNT CUT.

There are two spots, one on either side of the temple (above the outer ends of your brows), that for most people must be a bit longer because this hair has a tendency to recede and gets more wear and tear here than in any other place on your head. Something else to take into account when you are cutting hair: if you hair has any curve or curl in it at all, it will swing out in a spiral making your hair curve in on one side and curve out on the other. This is simply the way *everybody's* hair grows. When your hair is starting to get dry you might look at it and think that it's too short on one side, but before you cut, pull the hair out on either side of the face and visually measure it. If they are actually the same it is best not to cut anymore but to let the hair adjust to the cut for a couple of days. It takes at least this long for the hair to find its natural "bend" again and it should behave much better by then. Because the hair gets drier as you cut you can almost see the bend the hair is going to take and cut accordingly, but if the hair gets *too* dry on the ends, it should be re-wet slightly to make cutting more accurate.

Finally, comb all the hair out straight again and trim all around the original curve once more to even out the curve. With your head upside-down, shake the hair around again with your fingers and shape it by twisting it between your fingers and pulling it out away from gravity. Then just sit up and let it dry naturally. You may find a spot or two when it's dry that needs additional trimming. That's why I always leave my scissors out until I see what it looks like dry. Once it is *completely* dry you can brush through it, but this is up to you.

Cutting is really easy once you build up your confidence. The next time you get your hair cut, notice what your hairdresser does; you will hopefully see him using the techniques I've just talked about. If you would rather not cut hair, at least now you will be able to assess your hairdresser's style.

Most of your hair grooming you can do yourself, so let's start with a basic shampoo. I like to wash my hair in the shower where I can really rinse it clean after I shampoo. I pick a shampoo that has been pH balanced like one of Potions Eternal's many deliciously flavored shampoos or "Amino Pon" made by Redken labs. If you can't find a pH-balanced shampoo, it is best to stick to one of the milder, better brands which you are sure doesn't contain detergents that are too harsh for your hair. Many people like Johnson's Baby Shampoo because it is so mild. Whether you wash once or twice is up to you. When my hair feels very dirty I give it two sudsings, but this is very seldom since I wash my hair almost every day.

I was assured by one of New York's leading experts in hair treatment, Rita Hartinger, that daily washing is very healthy for the hair because it stimulates growth. Not only that, but I learned that very hot water is also good while shampooing because it stimulates circulation and the gland's production of natural oil.

She showed me that you get a bonus when you wash your hair and massage it at the same time because daily hair massage keeps it thick and healthy. As a matter of fact, this is one of the main things you can do for yourself to prevent thinning and falling hair and to stimulate new and *thicker* growth. My hair expert showed me a drawing of a cross-section of the scalp complete with hair folicles and all the different levels of the skin in which it grows.

With a healthy head of hair, the deep layer of skin from which the hair follicle grows is quite thick and spongy, thus giving the hair an ideal base—a kind of cushioned, well-nourished bed in which to grow. However, on examining the cross-section of someone with thinning hair, this same layer of tissue is noticeably less thick and spongy looking. I could easily see that the condition of the scalp makes the hair follicle itself grow either fat or skinny. It was obvious which came from which. The whole point of this is to stress, that by regularly massaging the scalp you too can have a thick, spongy bed in which to grow *your* hair!

Massaging is a snap to do: spread the finger tips over the head and press firmly on the scalp, making sure to push away all hair not growing on that spot. Gently rotate the scalp about the head in that spot until you feel well-massaged, then move on to the next one and the next one until you have pretty well covered your whole head.

If you really want to get into it, there's another massage evolving out of the first one that you can do. In this one you pull the finger tips of each hand toward one spot, grabbing the hair between your fingers and holding it firmly so that when you move your hand around in that spot, the captive hair *directly* moves the scalp beneath it. Grabbing the hair too far away from the scalp results in pulling the hair which hurts and could damage it. When you're doing it right it feels great. Do this all over your head until you've covered every inch.

If you were to massage your scalp gently for five minutes every day, the increased circulation and stimulation that result from doing it would reward you with a much thicker and healthier head of hair. I now do it automatically whenever my scalp feels tight and tense. Your scalp feels positively electric after a few minutes of massage and your hair looks great!

While I was learning this massage, I discovered something surprising about creme rinses. Rita Hartinger matter-of-factly explained to me that creme rinse tends to make your hair heavy and limp because of the sticky coating it forms around the shaft of each hair. "It is better," she said, "to use nothing at all." I'm sure there are times when you would disagree with her. When your hair is very long and in bad shape or if you have permed or bleached hair that is badly damaged, a conditioner may be the only solution for getting your hair combed out. However, if your hair is trimmed once every three or four weeks, a rinse is just a hindrance.

Trimming the hair this often is a *must* if you expect your hair to grow long and stay healthy looking. By continually snipping away split ends, you prevent them from getting tangled with and damaging the normal hairs. The chain reaction of breakage and split ends is stopped cold by scissors. If only the ends are snipped each time, more hair grows than is lost. Without trimming, the hair's growth is usually too slow to keep up with the breakage rate. If you've ever asked yourself "Why doesn't my hair *ever* grow?" this could be the answer.

So after you have washed your just trimmed hair, what do you do with it if you don't use a creme rinse? Nothing, if you use a pH-balanced shampoo. If you don't, some lemon juice dissolved in a cup of warm water will leave it glossy *and* acid-balanced nature's way.

After stepping out of the shower, if your hair isn't very long, you don't need to do any more than wrap it Turkish-style and leave it that way long enough to blot out the excess water, less than a minute.

To get your hair dry the natural way, bend over and shake your hair out with your fingers. This is done with a slapping, shaking motion of the fingers combined with loosening the hair around the scalp with the finger tips, making it almost dry in a minute or two.

If you have a good haircut, when you stand up your hair will fall out, almost away from the head, and will dry with all the natural body you were born with. Even if you think your hair is too curly or too straight to dry naturally, try doing it this way once and decide to like it for just a few minutes. That's the way I like it best anyway.

There are exceptions, of course. Sometimes I'm in the mood to curl it, sometimes to straighten it. There are so many ways to artificially dry hair to create different styles: You can use a curling iron; a dryer and brush; brush dry it; set it in hot rollers; set it in regular rollers and use a dryer or let it air dry; or set it in pin curls. And then you can always get a permanent too, which if done well can add curl and body if you like to have it curly all the time. I got my first permanent in years several months ago and *love* it!

Hair should *never* be forcibly brushed out when it is wet and tangled. I prefer starting with the head upside down. If a brush is used, it should be brushed a little at a time starting from the ends, holding and brushing just the bottom and working your way up to the scalp, never pulling and tugging. All this will keep the wet hair from overstretching and losing its elasticity or breaking.

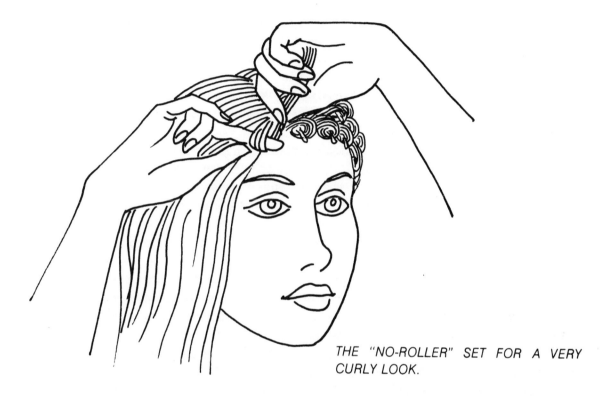

THE "NO-ROLLER" SET FOR A VERY CURLY LOOK.

I have a special way of setting my hair without any rollers: you start the curl close to the scalp and one layer at a time wrap the hair around your finger. When you remove your finger and stick a bobby pin straight through the lower part of the curl, the rest of it is standing straight up in the air as though it were wrapped around an invisible curler. The amount of hair in one curl doesn't usually cover more than a rectangle of scalp one inch by a half inch and is sometimes smaller (creating a very curly hairdo). If the curls get any bigger, drying it might require a blow or regular dryer.

Small curls dry in less than an hour. If you don't have the time to dry it completely and your hair is still slightly damp, take out the pins, bend over head down, and gently use the end of a rat-tail comb to loosen up the curls and bit by bit, fluff the hair out and away from the face. Then when you stand up again, the hair should stand way out and dry just right. If and when you brush and style it, try brushing upside down first and your hair will look so great that it won't even need styling.

By the way, my very favorite hair pins in the world, as far as I know, can only be found in one

beauty supply store in Los Angeles (and can be ordered in quantity from the manufacturer).*
This particular store caters mainly to the film industry. They are called "Blend-Rite ZIP
Finishing Pins." They are no-shine, tight and straight except for one crinkle in the middle;
have a narrow opening rubber tip; and are coated with a roughly textured, dull paint finish in
your choice of blond, brown, or black. They are great for a set because your slick, shiny hair
won't slip out like with other pins and can be used for finishing a hairdo when both nonslip and
no-shine qualities are required.

I set my hair this way almost exclusively. You can also set it the same way dry, using bigger
sections of hair. And after taking out the pins in the morning, a good massage and many
upside-down strokes will leave it looking fluffy and beautiful again. After letting your hair dry
naturally, you can brush it out by upside-down brushing and have it come out looking great.
This is just another form of massaging the scalp and increasing circulation.

One other way I occasionally set my hair is with a curling iron. This is tricky to learn to use
but well worth the effort. For beginners, the low heat and steam, teflon- or plastic-coated
curling irons are the safest. The metal kind must be handled very carefully for the sake of your
hair and your hands as they get quite hot. But they have the advantage of being more efficient
and are therefore faster.

Oh, there is another quick set that is great for longish hair: Part the hair, still slightly damp,
front to back; brush all the hair on one side into a large spiral curl and neatly pin it in three or
four places, taking care to avoid putting the hair in tension and making crimp marks; then do
the other side; leave it up for an hour or so (or overnight); and then use the upside-down and
fluffing-out hair technique.

I don't know if you noticed or not, but my favorite setting methods don't require any hair
dryers if you are reasonably patient. But a hair dryer is okay, set at a moderate heat, to speed
things up a bit when you're in a hurry or if you set your hair in rollers (the best kind are metal
coils covered with nylon netting). Sometimes in an emergency I use heated rollers but these
dry out the hair so they are only good for occasional use. A hand dryer to blow-dry the hair is
good for some styles and is the least damaging method of heated dryers.

If you are permanently coloring your hair, you probably know that bleaching is an integral
part of the process to keep color in. Bleaching makes the hair shaft less shiny and compact,
and more porous, this distortion being necessary to make the dye take. If you have extraordi-
narily thick hair, coloring it may even seem to improve the body, but in reality the hair has
been weakened. Coloring tends to make hair frizz rather than fall naturally.

If you color your hair yourself or have it done, keep a hawk's eye on the regrowth line and
make sure the touch-up color/bleach doesn't overlap the already bleached hair. This only
makes it lighter underneath the color and weaker yet, especially if you have fine hair.

If you have had it with bleaching and long to get your real hair back, you can let your own
hair grow out unobstrusively by getting a darker permanent color (one time only) to match
what yours will be when it grows out (remember your hair line is always considerably darker
than your grown-out hair because of exposure to sun and wear) and from then on, by getting
what they call a semi-permanent rinse which, although it won't continue to bleach your hair,
will rinse out after a few washings. When my hair was growing out I used one of the darker

*Sta-Rite Ginnie Lou, Inc. Shelbyville, Illinois 62565.

Born Blond semi-permanent rinses by Revlon. I never used those little crystals that you add to the color because nothing on the package said what they were. Even though the salespersons always swore that they weren't bleach, I couldn't be sure. With a rinse there is no way to prevent overlapping the new growth with color. If there was even a little bleach, the new hair would get it, too, which would have defeated the purpose of growing out my hair.

Although I know many people who have colored their hair for years and love it that way, for me it was just too much of a hassle to keep it up. In order to keep it in the best condition possible, I had to learn to do it myself at home. Any overlap of the color/bleach would overly weaken my baby fine hair. Plus, hairdressers invariably would leave the bleach on for much longer than necessary which also weakens the hair (five minutes is enough time for my dark blond hair; one hour is sometimes necessary on other heads of hair).

I had colored my hair for so long that I had forgotten what my real color actually looked like. When it finally grew out I was delighted to see that it was a beautiful, dark ash blond and I looked better than I had in years. This is also when I started to realize that my hair had a little natural curl.

One alternative to total hair color is to get fine blond streaks put in your hair. If you can find an extremely conscientious hairdresser to do it very subtly and so that when it grows out it will only extend the blond that has already been done, then I would recommend it. Bad streaking jobs are what started me bleaching my hair in the first place: Pretty soon there was nothing left to streak!

The best way of all to give your hair sunny highlights is to lightly brush the bleach mixture just on the ends and gradually fade it in toward the scalp, making sure to touch only the top layer of hair. That way you never have to retouch roots and the highlights remain looking completely natural.

Permanents also weaken hair although they are done so well these days that there is no danger of damaging the hair if you have a hairdresser you can trust. The only danger arises when your hair is already bleached or colored and you decide you want it permed too or vice versa. This is asking for trouble. Be sure to check with your hairdresser so he can test your hair first. Redken Laboratories will analyze a hair strand for you and tell you whether or not your hair can take a perm.

Heated rollers or steam rollers are an alternative to permanents although if used too often, they can make your hair dry and brittle. If you are already using heated rollers or if you plan to, I suggest buying the conditioning spray made expressly for this purpose (for example, Clairol's Kindness, Heat-Activated Conditioner) and give your hair a once over with it before each setting for protection from dryness.

Although I don't recommend creme rinses, I do think an occasional conditioning is very good for the hair, especially if it is subjected to the frequent use of curling irons, heated rollers, back-combing, hairsprays, etc., that most models go through daily. There is such a variety of conditioners on the market that do so many different things that I can't recommend any one although I am partial to the ones that build up the hair shaft by filling in the porous parts of the hair with protein like Climatress by Redken. Some conditioners work best with a heat cap to penetrate the hair shaft more deeply. Others you can do yourself at home and leave on for fifteen minutes to overnight. You can even mash up a ripe avocado, massage it into your hair, and leave it on for an hour or so to soften and condition dry hair.

Even better for your hair than conditioners are the very new protein restructurers which are now available at beauty salons and from beauty supply houses. These, unlike the standard conditioners, do not coat the hair strand's exterior but actually go into the cortex of the hair and restructure and recondition the damaged molecules. The hair strand is actually so improved that the difference can be seen under a microscope. Redken produces microscopes and stress machines to determine the condition and strength of hair.

Victor of Configuro Salon in New York is one hairdresser who is interested in continually improving his client's hair and he uses these machines to determine just what treatment is needed.

Naturally some products are better than others. For example, Jhirmack's hydrolized protein, called N.C.A., uses the R.N.A. factor in amino acids which "orders" the protein into greater compatibility with hair. Besides Jhirmack, Victor might use Redken's P.P.T., a hydrolized protein product which binds to the already existing protein in the hair, or Extreme which also contains citric acid and lipids for moisture-starved hair. Sometimes he works just with organic products like honey, aloe, nettle, eggs, avocado, or banana extract and sometimes combinations of different organic and commercial substances. Victor feels that Loreal's Inerol is a good product for rebuilding hair structure. As a moisturizing agent he recommends Redken's Climatress and Jhirmack's Nutripack which not only contains the excellent protein restructurers found in N.C.A. but has, in addition, humicants (moisturizers) which are good for treating more extreme damage.

If you are a sun and sports enthusiast like so many Californians, you should definitely take measures to protect your hair from the sun and the wind. Sometimes I saturate my hair with conditioner, pull it back with a covered band, and tuck the tail into a bun before I go out for private sunbathing. The easily burned ends of the hair are protected and the hair around the face can get nature's lightening from the sun. If you are in a place where you don't want to be seen with your hair slathered with conditioner or if you are going to be swimming a lot, then you should wear a hat or a scarf while you are sunning.

Hats or scarves are a *must* for open-air sports driving or boating if you want any hair left at all at the end of a summer. If you can't find a hat or a scarf, then at least pull your hair back in a band.

Wearing your hair pulled tightly back in a band all the time is definitely not good for the hair or for your head. It can cause your hair to grow thinner and can pull out hair as well as causing breakage. Continual tension on your scalp sometimes causes headaches and baldness. I get the covered bands made especially for pony tails to protect the hair and reduce tension.

About the only other thing I can think of that you should protect your hair from is yourself. You may unknowingly be causing damage several ways. When combing or brushing you have to be very gentle, especially if you have fine hair, so that you don't break it. If you have tangles, start from the bottom and brush or comb a little at a time, gradually working your way up to the hair at the top. Work patiently with each tangle to break as little hair as possible. This care is even more important when your hair is wet because excessive pulling will stretch the hair's natural bounce right out and leave it thin and lifeless looking until it is replaced by new hair.

There is one other area in which you should be wary, but if you are not a model you probably will never experience this problem. Some hairdos require back-combing, back-brushing, and hair spray to get them to stand out and stay there. This in itself isn't too bad, but afterward when the hair is combed out you have to be extremely careful and patiently comb out each individual section of hair. I have seen hairdressers whack out the back combing with a brush with no regard for the poor girl who has to wake up the next day with broken hair. And she may not even realize how it got that way!

In summary, if you keep your hair washed almost daily and trimmed every few weeks and do as little to it as possible except protect it from the sun and wind, and if you eat well and get plenty of exercise, you should have a head full of beautiful, shiny, vibrant hair.

Makeup

Makeup is many things to many different people. Models and movie stars have to wear so much makeup so often that they welcome the chance to be as natural as possible and wear the unmadeup look. They feel secure enough around their friends to drop their image for awhile and be themselves. I don't mean they wear no makeup at all. Even the most secure beauties I know wear a little makeup when they aren't in the spotlight because they still want to look beautiful, and since no one is perfect, they have to work with this or that flaw or maybe use something to bring out their eyes.

When I am not working in public and am in and around my home environment, I try to let my image stand to the side by wearing no makeup at all. That way I am my most open, sensitive, and vulnerable, which is the way I like to be. But on a day that I feel a bit insecure or just not very beautiful, I go discreetly to my bag of makeup tricks and put on just enough to make me feel beautiful in the accepted sense.

Sometimes I resent having to wear makeup because I am a naturalist at heart. I am most comfortable taking in the sun and waves on a South Sea island and wearing absolutely nothing at all. When I am relaxed and close to nature my complexion is so good that I don't even have to think about putting on makeup.

I sometimes fantasize about a futuristic society with people having no hang-ups, men and women absolutely equal, and clothes and makeup relics of an ancient past. But back in the city and faced with the reality of day-to-day living, makeup is indeed a boon. Sometimes it is an absolute necessity to escape into the make-believe, real world of movies, rock stars, models, presidents, executives, society, foreign intrigue, or whatever.

If it catches your fancy at the moment, you can put on any of those images in makeup and act out the part just for the fun of it. Wouldn't it be boring if we couldn't change our dress and makeup to suit our many different moods?

So with this in mind I invite you to enjoy the fantasy-reality of "putting on a face." I encourage you to change and experiment, be subtle or daring, be Cleopatra or Alice in Wonderland. But no matter what role you decide to enact, always remember who you really are and let your beautiful self come shining through.

Whenever I give someone a makeup lesson I generally encourage her to be as natural as possible because most women tend to be heavy handed with makeup.

Day makeup is generally softer and lighter than night, so if you keep this in mind I will take you step-by-step through a complete "ready for anything" makeup.

Now is a good time to mention that if you expect to do a competent makeup job, proper lighting is a *must!* I prefer putting on makeup to be worn for the day in sunlight which comes from directly behind me (light from directly in front also works if it is not too bright). Side light is disastrous for making up because you really can't match one side of your face to the other. If sunlight isn't available when you put on your makeup and you expect to go out into the sun later, carry a small mirror with you so that you can make adjustments if necessary. I find that the cheeks are almost always too red when switching from artificial light to sunlight.

For artificial lighting situations or for night the best makeup light comes from incandescent light placed just above your mirror or slightly above and ahead. Lights around the sides and the top of your mirror are ideal if their combined effect is not too bright, but this situation is a rare pleasure even for a model. Fluorescent lights are murder for makeup. You can stand there and put on makeup forever and still think you look ugly because this kind of light picks up the blue in your veins directly below the top layer of skin and any other imperfections. If the only fixtures available are set up for fluorescent lighting, either move or change the fixtures, but in the meantime use "warm light" tubes as they are the best you can do immediately. In some cities you can buy the new "Vita Light" fixtures, which have the best color balance for skin. The fixtures are manufactured by Duro Test of New Jersey.

Before you start your hands and face should be clean, but the face should not be too freshly washed as the pores should have a chance to be tightly closed before you start. You should already be wearing something to protect your face, either a moisturizer or a toner depending on whether your skin is dry or oily. If your face looks oily from too much moisturizer, you can use a kleenex, facial blotting papers, or perhaps your hands to blot off the excess oil until your face has a natural dewy finish.

Basically this is the way it will stay, too, because I never recommend using a base. Using a base simply means that you cover your entire face with a one-color, thin film of makeup. In real life even the most beautiful, flawless complexions are never all one color and tone so if natural, beautiful skin is what you strive to achieve with makeup, you can forego the base completely. A base might be an exception if you have freckles and you don't want them to show. But personally I love freckles and if I had them they would be right out there in the open, unabashedly exposed.

If you insist on using a base, the water-based hypo-allergenic ones are best for oily skin and a light, slightly or nonoily kind is best for normal to dry skins. Definitely avoid the greasy or thick kinds, pan stick and pancake makeup. These are all right for stage or TV but are not good for your skin for prolonged periods of time. Remember that your skin must breathe if it is to be healthy.

Because I rarely wear a base and have never been allergic to anything, I buy any brand of makeup that has the right color and texture that I seek. But if you have ever been allergic to cosmetics or if you have sensitive skin and want to do it a favor, stick to the hypo-allergenic brands of makeup. The major brands include Clinique by Estee Lauder, Ethera by Revlon, Almay by Schefflein and Co., and R X Company products. There are others, too, but you will have to ask and check labels for these. There are many organic makeups available, too; these are probably better for you, if you can find the colors and textures that you like.

The first thing I do (since I don't use a base and my face is properly protected with moisturizer) is put a little color in my cheeks and accentuate my cheek bones. If you have difficulty in deciding the intensity of color you wish to use, pick your lipstick first to somewhat match what you plan to wear and first put a bit of color on your mouth for color balance which you will finish later.

Several things can be used for the cheeks. For day or more casual makeup I like to use a pinkish gel. It takes a while to learn to apply this evenly and to fade the edges into your skin, but it feels so clean that it's worth the trouble. You must spread it quickly with one or two gentle finger tips, completing and blending each section as you move on because it is almost impossible to go back unless you want to start over again. Before you start, *smile,* and apply color to the resulting ball of your cheek, bringing the color up along your cheekbone and out into your hairline. By the way, gel is *not* the best thing for oily complexions. A good alternative would be blush-on-type powders or creme rouge. Blot your face first with facial blotting papers to remove any excess oils.

For a more extreme makeup look I go to a dark rose pan stick for under the cheekbone (carefully blended into the hairline around the corner) and a red or pink rouge for the ball of the cheek when smiling and for the upper part of the cheekbone. Here it is important to blend the two colors carefully, both with each other and with the adjoining natural skin. There is nothing more distracting to me than a makeup that stops at the chin, or goes almost to the hair and suddenly stops, or any other abrupt patch of color or hard line in the makeup. Use a two-way mirror if you have to and remember good lighting.

Some people are happy to just use a brush-on-blusher in a pink to pink/brown shade which is alright, too, if you don't plan to wear any makeup over it. I do, however, find powder a bit drying on my skin. The powder always comes last in making up. To give blusher set with powder a more natural finish, gently blot your cheeks with a damp kleenex.

Before I go on to the next step, you should know about using shading to make a prominent area recede. This is best used for theatrical occasions because continuous use of makeup on your face can ruin your skin. To narrow a nose, put a little dark makeup (dark rose or a light brown pan stick) on either side of the nose. To make a protruding nose recede, use a slightly darker shade of makeup just along the length of the top. To narrow or make a prominent jaw bone recede, use a darker makeup along the jaw line. Generally speaking, receding features which you wish to bring out, make slightly lighter, and prominent features that you wish to make recede, make slightly darker.

If you decide to use this technique, be sure to make it look natural by blending it well with adjacent skin and rounding the corners that are out of your sight but seen by others. Too light or too dark makeup can make you look like a clown so don't defeat your own purpose by overdoing it! Wait until your entire makeup is done to powder because once the makeup is set, it is pretty hard to change effectively.

After the cheeks are done, but before using powder, is the best time to touch up blemishes and other not quite perfect features. The only time that I use cover-up makeup is when there is something I absolutely *have* to hide. If I have been eating well, exercising, and I'm feeling great, there is usually very little of this required. One of the cover-up areas might be dark circles under the eyes for which I use Geminesse eye-shadow cream, Sunlight #25 by Max Factor, dotted on very lightly with just the top of a finger. (If you are not fair, the shade you pick should be just slightly lighter than your skin.) This makeup is water-based and although it contains a little oil, it must be spread quickly but carefully. Don't try a second coat as this will ruin the first. It would be better for touching up over the first coat to use a makeup brush to dab on just the faintest amount of pan-stick makeup a hair lighter than your natural shade; then lightly powder over this.

I keep three, long-handled sable makeup brushes about ¼ inch by ½ inch with the hairs of the brush gently tapered: one for dark colored oil-based makeup, one for light colored oil-based makeup, and one for dark water-based makeup. This may seem like a lot of trouble, but mixing colors and opposing bases on one brush can keep you very busy cleaning if you don't want to spoil your makeup job. The same is generally true of mixing opposing bases on your face but there are several exceptions, the above being one of them because with a little practice you can sometimes make it work.

Other touch-up areas would be discolorations, moles, pimples, etc., which you simply dot lightly with the same pan-stick brush used above. Pat the spot gently with the very tip of a finger until it seems to blend in with the adjoining skin. Two makeup applications are sometimes necessary. Then lightly tap on a bit of powder from a small powder brush to set the makeup and give it an unobtrusive matt-finish. (For powdering I use about a 4-inch handle brush with sable hairs ¾ inches long by ⅜ by ⅛ inches and with the end gently tapered.) If you have a particularly obstinate spot to cover up you can apply, *very carefully,* a second coat of makeup with just the tip of the brush, pat gently, and powder again. This almost always does the trick.

I use loose, transparent, natural-colored face powder. This can be used to set spots that you are touching up, or once again, when your makeup job is finished, to lightly powder your entire face. Overall powdering should be done with a fat, round-shaped sable brush. This, however, is a step I rarely use because I don't normally wear a base. In my small makeup bag that travels with me on all my assignments I carry only a scant amount of powder which I put in a smaller container that I once got as a powder sample. As a matter of fact, I do this with all of my makeup that comes in large or bulky containers, thus saving a lot of space and weight to carry around. If you are smart, a see-through plastic makeup bag with a zipper (about 12 by 6 by 2 inches) should easily hold all the makeup you will ever have to use.

To get back to the makeup job at hand: You now have most of your face under control so the next area to go to is the eyes. A basic eye makeup for me starts by using a dark grease pencil or brown grease crayon (from Mary Quant's coloring box) all around the eyes as close to the lashes as you can get. Make it narrow and light on the bottom and inside corners and thicker and darker on the top. Then above the crease line's natural crescent, I start at the inside corner and make a one-quarter-inch-wide stroke with the crayon, following the shape of the crescent, and continue the line at the end of the eye out and up toward the hairline another quarter inch. Above this color I use a pinker-than-flesh-tone pink crayon into which I blend the brown. I fill in the lower part of the upper lid (just below the crescent) with whatever color appeals to me at the moment, perhaps matching what I am wearing. I might choose pink or light blue for day and gold for night for example. Then I carefully blend this color into the brown of the crescent above and into the line next to the upper lashes below. After blending, if the brown liner above the upper lashes is too faded, I darken the line with more brown. The faint brown line just under the lower lashes I soften with my finger tip so you hardly know it's there.

Brown is a good, basic eyeliner color for light complexions and the darker your skin, the blacker this line can be. Some people prefer a liquid eyeliner but this is much more difficult to blend with other colors and to make subtle enough to look natural. Powders for the upper lid are another choice, but here too it is difficult to blend colors and get just the intensity you like. On me, it also tends to make my eyes dry and crinkly looking.

I use colors around the eyes when I am bored with brown. A purple liner and accent above the crease line blended into violet and then rose is an example of a more dramatic effect. A completely radical eye makeup that is great for colorful summer parties is to make a rainbow of colors starting from the inside corner of your eye and gradually, blending one color into the next, adding perhaps violet, red, orange, yellow, and green.

The important thing to remember when doing your eyes is to use colors and shades as though you were an artist gently blending colors with the balls of your fingers. Oily-based cremes or crayons are perfect for this purpose. If you prefer, you can apply the colors with a one-quarter-inch-wide makeup brush. If the colors don't go on smoothly, add a dot or two of vitamin E from the capsule to lubricate. If your eyes are deep set, use lighter shades to bring them out and forgo the dark line above the crease. If your eyes need depth then the darker shades are appropriate. Under no circumstances should you actually see any lines when you have completed your eyes, unless you want to look like a clown.

If, after you have had your "eyes on" for awhile, you tend to collect some color in the crease, you can use a Kleenex around the tip of your finger to absorb the excess makeup without ruining your eye makeup if you are careful.

Applying mascara is the last step for the eyes. How carefully you apply it will make or break the success of your eye-makeup job, so take your time and do it right. I use a brown brush-on wand mascara. If you have very dark skin you should use black (colored mascaras are fun for special occasions). Start by blotting the tip of the wand on a Kleenex to remove the extra goop that has accumulated there so it won't all end up on one spot on your lashes. Starting at the inside corner of your upper lashes, make a few delicate strokes from the base of the lashes on out to almost the tip, concentrating on the area nearest the base.

Rather than getting it perfect the first time, continue out toward the outside corner of the eye, using several strokes for each section as you go along. Then, replace the wand in the applicator tube once, blot the tip again, and do the same thing with the upper lashes of the other eye starting at the inside corner and working your way out.

The next is a very important step: With a tiny comb made especially for eyelashes and eyebrows (found at beauty supply stores or a well-equipped drugstore), carefully comb the mascara through the lashes to separate any lashes which may have stuck together or gotten much mascara in one spot. This will even out the first application and give your lashes a first appl... look. You should do this before the mascara dries. If you find that applying the comb the mascara upper lashes of both eyes takes too long, and by the time you use the one eye, blot the comb on dry, then only do one eye at a time. When you are through with

Repeat the above process on the x before going to the next eye. attention as the upper ones but much less lashes which require just as much time and

Survey the almost finished effect in your mirror. I y... for a softer-finished eye. mascara, apply this one much lighter than the first, once again li...tly separating lashes with the comb if necessary. Continue the stroke all the way out to the tips of the lashes and with the tip of a finger, whisk away the excess mascara on the tips of the lashes for a softer, more natural look. This also keeps the mascara from transferring over to the upper or lower eyelid.

And finally, all you should have left to do is to finish your lips which you may have started in the beginning by adding a bit of color as a guide.

There are several effective ways to do lips, the choice of which depends on your mood or preference. I generally pick a dark-brown rose (not too creamy) and quickly but sparingly fill in the inside portions, pressing my lips together to spread the lipstick evenly. Then I carefully draw the outer line all the way around my lips either with a lip brush or with the lipstick itself if I am in a hurry, making sure to accent the peaks and to fill in the corners of the mouth. I then blot with a Kleenex by opening my mouth wide, inserting the Kleenex between upper and lower lips, and blotting down with the mouth one time only, smiling slightly to take up the excess in any cracks. On your Kleenex there should be the shape of perfect lips if you did it right. I dot on a drop or two of vitamin E in the center to make the inside of the lips moist but the outer lip line firm.

Another method is to draw the outer line first with a brown grease pencil made especially for this purpose and then fill in with your favorite color. The brown line almost disappears but accents your lip line enough to make your lips look full and sexy.

You can do the same with a lip brush using a not-too-creamy color to line in a darker shade and then fill in the inner portions of the mouth with a creamier, lighter or brighter color. The reason I don't use a creamy color for a lip line is because the oils in this type of lipstick "bleed" easily and end up making fuzzy lines past your lip line that really look ridiculous. To prevent this you can line your lips first, blot gently with a tissue, powder lightly with a brush, and then fill in the mouth with a creamy color. This helps maintain the shape of the outer lips even through a meal. I only do this for special occasions, though, as it tends to be a bit drying.

Now you should have a finished, natural looking makeup. When you are all through, examine the overall effect and make sure that everything is evenly balanced. Sometimes it is necessary to brush on a bit more powder or use blotter papers if there are any shiny spots. Or perhaps add to or subtract from the makeup you've already put on.

Although I have taken you step-by-step through all the methods of application, I cannot teach you how to be an artist, which is what you become when you really do a good makeup job. If you feel insecure about how your makeup should look, try going through all the fashion magazines popular with your age group and tear out pictures of different makeups you like and try to duplicate them. After you have practiced a few times you should be more confident about doing your own experiments with colors and textures and find a good, basic make technique with which you feel comfortable. Pay attention to details and don't be s   which is it looks just right to you. Then no one will notice your makeup, they will n what you really wanted all along, isn't it?